GOODBYE STRESS, HELLO HAPPINESS

A PATH TO PEACE AND LOVE

Carol Ann Hontz

Publishing Company: Carol Ann Hontz International, Inc.

Copyright © 2008 by Carol Ann Hontz

First printing, February, 2009

Editors: Catherine Knowles and Gerald Kellett
Photographers: Tropical Imaging (Book Cover),
Timea Jakse (Photo of Carol Ann Hontz)

ISBN: 978-0-9822651-0-9

Printed in the United States of America

CONTENTS

Also by Carol Ann Hontz

Infinite Potential
Inner Treasures

The above may be ordered by visiting:

www.carolannhontz.com

DEDICATION

THIS book is lovingly dedicated to all our family of humanity. The healing process is real and an easy skill to develop. My trust is that the healing within each heart will burst the bonds of limitation, replacing them with peace, love, abundance, success, empowerment, vibrant health and great joy as seen in my clients' and students' lives. May all of humanity say goodbye stress, hello happiness!

IN APPRECIATION

I wish to thank the outstanding specialized kinesiologists and practitioners of natural, alternative healing modalities, who have devoted their lives to the facilitation of the healing process for themselves and others. From them, I have learned a whole new way of life in my service to humanity. These individuals have stood as strong as sturdy oak trees in the face of adversity in creating a bridge between the traditional methods and the alternative natural ways of healing and living. Many of these brave pioneers have passed on, but they remain in our hearts as some of the greatest unsung heroes of our modern times. They had the courage and fortitude to stand up for what they believed, in spite of great obstacles. They were successful long before machines could prove the effects in the body of a single thought. They have created systems so effective that it has changed millions of lives. They have facilitated the surfacing of that inner peace, calm and love, our main goal for the world. It is a rewarding experience to witness the ability of individuals to metamorphose their lives so gently, non-invasively and emerge as the beautiful beings they really are! My eternal gratitude goes to all of my dear teachers: Daniel Whiteside, Gordon Stokes, Anneke Kruit, Frank Mahoney, Dr. Wayne Topping, Dr. George Goodheart. Dr. Paul Dennison, Dr. John Thie, and Dr. Sheldon Diehl.

> "The potential of the average person is like a huge ocean unsailed,
> a new continent unexplored, a world of possibilities waiting to be
> released and channeled toward some great good."
>
> --Brian Tracy

SYNOPSIS OF CHAPTERS

Chapter 1 Fear: Fear paralyzes the individual and the world. We were not born with most fears; they were programmed in, usually at a very early age. Fear controls most of our behaviors today. Many fears are listed, with their gentle, easy, effective, lasting corrections given. Following are a few specific examples of fears that are addressed in the first chapter: fear of flying, ladders/heights, public speaking, authority, and people.

Chapter 2 Emotional Pain: "Pain is a sensation, a perception, an emotion, cognition, a motivation and it is energy, in sum, a highly integrated, multifaceted phenomenon," said Dr. David E. Bresler. Emotional pain prompts physical pain and physical pain prompts emotional pain. This chapter shows examples of how the cause of emotional pain was identified and thus corrected. Some examples are: panic attacks, parental rejection, anger, suicidal tendencies, eating disorders, road rage, and depression.

Chapter 3 Physical Pain: As stated before, emotional and physical pain can be a vicious cycle. When we clear the emotional pain, the physical body can heal itself very quickly, sometimes instantly. In this chapter are cases where the emotional pain was corrected; consequently, physical pain symptoms could vanish. Clients have corrected the meridian energy flow and thus the symptoms could disappear in areas such as: arthritis pain, pain in various parts of the body (back, limbs, head, and neck), high blood pressure, enlarged prostate, skin problems, exhaustion, burping, and accidents.

Chapter 4 Relationships: Relationships are one of the most problematic areas of our lives. These include primary relationships, family, colleagues, friends, and business relationships. Wars are created at home, in classrooms, in offices, on streets, and among nations. Why? It goes back to an individual and his/her lack of inner peace. We do not love ourselves because someone told us we were not perfect and not lovable. We did not meet their standard for behavior. Sadly, we believed their evaluation of us. This chapter deals with the following interactions and some of their solutions: open, direct communication, listening, telling the truth, expressing our viewpoints and accepting others (although we may not agree), recognizing equality and our inner truth. The following relationships are categorized and examples of corrections given: child/parent in specific times such as prenatal, birth, early childhood (the most formative years), student/teacher relationships, personal relationships and relationships in social responsibility areas.

Chapter 5 Sexual Challenges: Countless sexual problems today are caused by molestation at a very early age, often by a family member. This chapter highlights that cause (as well as others) and corrections of deep sexual problems, in such areas as sexual satisfaction, ability to conceive, male and female organ malfunction, hormone imbalances, birthing problems, and compulsive behavioral problems. The goal of this information is to let individuals know that there is help to re-establish self-esteem and therefore feelings of self-worth in being a male or female and healing the emotional body. Each one must forgive himself/herself and the other person involved for healing to take place. As in other chapters, representative examples are given.

Chapter 6 Learning Challenges: Many learning problems can be corrected when we address the root cause: stress. When stress is present in a learning situation and the individual is overwhelmed, a survival pattern is set up which programs in a blind spot. For example, when an individual is 30 years old, he does not remember that embarrassing, traumatic situation in third grade with numbers and doesn't know why he is blocked in mathematics, but the stress remains. Until we release the emotional pain from that deeply buried memory, the individual is not in control and will repeat that same pattern. Included in this chapter is my research with 80 students in the school for the learning-impaired in Budapest and the results. Some learning challenge examples addressed here are with reading, writing, mathematics, hearing, speaking, vision, logic, creativity, physical balance as well as left/right balance of the brain hemispheres.

Chapter 7 Allergies: When stress is present, for example, at the time we are eating a certain food, smelling a specific odor, or cutting the lawn, we can associate that food, odor, person, location, etc. with a feeling of rejection of self or others. This can set up an allergic reaction to that substance, situation, condition, person or place. The allergy examples corrected in this chapter are to: milk, fish, fragrances, weather, hot peppers, onions, plants, and paint. By correcting the emotion that created that allergy, we correct the cause of the allergy and thus the symptoms.

Chapter 8 Compulsive Behavior: Most major fears are programmed in by age six. If we do not correct these fears, they become our addictions to keep us living in present time, feeling as good as we possibly can. We do not want to remember the fear and pain of the past, so we stay numb with drugs, alcohol, cigarettes, etc. If we do not handle these addictions, they become our obsessions in the future--obsessed with the thought of having enough alcohol, sex, drugs, of being in a certain location, with a certain person, etc. Some examples addressed in this chapter are compulsive behaviors relating to objects, alcohol, drugs, smoking, over-eating, procrastination, indecision, sleeping, failure, autism, perfectionism and attachments. Compulsive behaviors encompass mental, physical, emotional and spiritual fears as well as addictions and obsessions.

Chapter 9 Death and Dying: Most people have much stress on these two areas with a fear that they will have a long, painful, expensive end and then -- what follows? How we feel about death now will help to determine how we will eventually face it. If we accept our own mortality with grace as part of the human cycle, then our adjustments will be much easier. It is the quality of our lives that is important, not the length. Elizabeth Kubler-Ross stated that when people are dying, they regret two things: they did not tell someone they loved them and they did not live out their life's dream. When working on this issue with clients, for example, I ask them what it is that they would like to tell that person who has left them. I ask them what they imagine that person would now say back to them. We may also work with forgiveness, often a major issue. In this chapter, I relate my personal experience of my son's departing several years ago, including the coincidences surrounding that. We may accept that our departed loved ones are in their perfect place and that we will one day be also.

Chapter 10 Forgiveness, Love and Peace: If we hold onto anger, resentment and are unforgiving, it has a toxic effect on our bodies. The body produces stress hormones for a certain situation in order to survive, but when that event is over, the body can still hold the stress until we re-pattern it. By information and examples, this chapter helps us to understand that we may not agree with or understand someone's motives for behaving as they do, but under the circumstances, they are doing the best they know how, given their early life programming. Highlighted are the major religious groups' principles concerning forgiveness. A trauma surgeon gives his testimony on forgiveness before his passing. The final area of this chapter deals with the area of love, the highest goal and vibration. When we love ourselves, we can then accept and even love others.

FOREWORD

EIGHTEEN years have elapsed since the publication of my first book, "Infinite Potential". Years add to our knowledge, experience and expertise. However, the basic conditions, human characteristics, and motivating forces behind humankind have not changed very much. Wherever I travel, the basic theme of love, acceptance and peace are what people really desire deep down in their souls. These years have taken me to Russia, Hungary, The Czech and Slovak Republics and Poland. In the early 1990's, these countries were eager for new ways to approach the problems of life with hope and trust in a new future. I have had the exceptional pleasure of working with thousands of students and clients who were looking for and ready for a better way, a more healthful, happier, more creative way of life. They have found it through our work together.

It is now my desire to share with my readers, the details of how lives have been changed easily, quickly and non-invasively for the better, and in major ways!

The challenges of the world weigh much greater on its citizens today than at any other time in history. I have great faith that countless numbers of average individuals, who amaze me with their capabilities, will supply the world with the solutions needed. We must solve the enormous problems of today in the areas of health, education, energy, environment, government, finances, food, clothing, shelter, security. The solutions are only waiting to be recognized and implemented.

At times we may feel overwhelmed with the problems of the world. If each one of us does his/her part in making the world a better place, then based on the principle of "The Hundredth Monkey", we shall solve the problems together. So many people today are lonely, feel loveless or unlovable. Peace and love is their quest. If "average" people can develop a happier and healthier life, then what can we do for the depressed, discouraged person? This book will tell you!

We are a totality of "be-ing". It is impossible to separate the body, mind, emotions and spirit to classify and categorize. However, for practical modern references, I have divided the chapters into specific categories and some into sub-categories. Please realize that all facets of life are intertwined and inseparable.

How does this method of specialized kinesiology work? Our model differs from the medical model in that we work on the energy field and not specifically on the physical body. In 1964, Dr. George Goodheart discovered that when he put certain substances on the body and tested a muscle, the energy given off by the substance caused the muscle to either hold strong or to weaken. Later it was discovered that when thinking of a specific event or word, that thought or word alone could either strengthen or weaken the muscles of the body, depending on what were the individual's feelings about that event or thought.

Five thousand years ago, the Chinese learned that energy travels along energy flow lines called meridians. Acupuncturists use meridians in their work. The body energy is disturbed when any thought, emotion, or the environment causes a stress reaction, therefore a blockage in the meridian system.

With stress testing we can discover when, where and how that disturbance occurred and how to redirect the energy by way of very gentle, non-invasive techniques. We do not cure disease. We balance the energy of the individual; then, the body does a wonderful job of rejuvenating itself, sometimes instantly!

When a person has a desire to be healed, the facilitator assists in balancing the energy with the "body intelligence". It is the person's body that does the healing. Deepak Chopra stated, "To promote the healing response, you must get past all the grosser levels of the body -- cells, tissue, organs, and systems and arrive at a junction between mind and matter, the point where consciousness actually starts to have an effect."

As I work through issues with my clients and students, the

realizations they must reach are deep in the emotional body. There the focus is one of forgiving themselves and others and then loving themselves and accepting others. Healing happens with love and acceptance. Each of us has love deeply buried within us. When we remove the layers of a lifetime of fear and pain, love is brought to the surface for each of us, even the most hardened criminals.

I am not a "healer". I just show people how to heal themselves. I facilitate their healing. It can happen very quickly when they are ready. We simply identify the issue that is causing stress in their lives. Then, go to the first original cause/age of that stress through biofeedback and release the pain in that memory. Finally, it may remain just a memory but without that stressful pain previously associated with it.

The process is so gentle and non-invasive with simple exercises to restore the meridian energy flow and balance the body/brain. Clients and students are then asked how their life will be different if they no longer have stress on the issue controlling them. They take back their power and become more of who they really are with each layer of stress removed. The cases mentioned in this book are but a small fraction of the cases which I have felt honored to facilitate. They occurred primarily in the former Soviet Union and Eastern European countries where fear, pain, lack of freedom and war were such a major part of their existence for many decades. Through this process people feel as though they have emerged from a dark, closed period of their lives. You too can emerge from any dark times and transform yourself into the happy, peaceful, loving being we were all intended to be!

For numerous examples in the book from recent years, I asked the students' and clients' permission to use their stories. They were happy to be in the book and said I could use their names. However, I have decided not to include their names in case that, in the future, they may be in a situation where they would not want that information to be public. I thank them from the bottom of my heart for the sharing of their personal experiences to help others.

CHAPTER 1

FEAR

FEARS attach themselves to us like barnacles. They are not really a part of us, but a belief system which we acquired because of our feelings from a past traumatic event. That belief system is held in the body as a thought and retains the energy that we give it. If a person says s/he is afraid of dogs, the more deeply ingrained the fear, the greater the fear reaction to dogs. If you are afraid of dogs and you talk often about this fear, you may reinforce it. Whatever you focus on is what you will have more of in your life!

~

If only we realized how much one single fear limits us. I recently worked with a client who had a great fear of spiders. She had just returned from a lovely vacation, but related that they had to move from their hotel because she had found a spider in their room. It was not only expensive to move, but what guarantee did she have that she would not encounter another spider in the next hotel?

As I was stress releasing her fear, we created a humorous situation about the spider and his spider-family so that she would have a more relaxed feeling about the creature. She considered the worst thing that could happen, perhaps a bite and medical attention, which would probably never occur. When I asked her how it would change her life if she no longer feared spiders, she replied that it would open all kinds of doors. For her, those doors that were closed down since a very early age are now open.

If a fear is always in the back of one's mind, then there is no peace. The person then expects more "spiders", for example, to be lurking around every corner.

~

The following client had the longest list of fears that I had ever encountered. Her outward appearance was that of a confident, capable business woman. She was about to be married and go on a safari honeymoon to Africa. The list of fears she brought to me seemed endless: the fear of fear, fear of pregnancy, of giving birth, being alone, money, ghosts, disease, death, flying, darkness, being unattractive, aging, insects (especially mosquitoes), speeding cars, vaccinations, chemicals, heights, new places, vacations, the unknown.

During the first private session with me, she added to the list: compulsive buying to cheer herself up, varicose veins, hearing loss, superstitions, irregular heartbeat, choking sensation, depression, panic attacks, anger with self, acne scars, back-aches, wedding preparation, feuding, divorced parents at the wedding, inside tremors when she doesn't eat on time.

To my astonishment and hers, by the end of the third session, we had solved most of the problems and deleted most of her fears!

Weeks later, she showed me her wedding and honeymoon photos -- so relaxed and happy, radiant throughout the whole wedding and trip. Flying was not a problem and the mosquitoes behaved nicely! She is a new person, or -- the real person she was underneath all the fear, pain and fear of pain. Hers was a profound metamorphosis!

Note: Two years later, this lady became the mother of a healthy, happy little girl who will not have the former fears of her mother transferred to her as so often occurs. We spend years building up the armor against fear and it can be released so gently and easily through the specialized kinesiology methodology.

~

If we look deeply into the problems of today's world, we will find that they are fear-based: the Oklahoma City bombings, Columbine

School shootings, and 9-11. What do they all have in common? The perpetrators were acting out of fear. Was it from fear of non-acceptance by society, fear that they as humans were not good enough? Was it fear of more rejection and emotional pain? What causes people to want to destroy another's life and even to take their own lives?

One tragedy after another has caused the American public to live in fear. What we cannot trust, we fear. Fear of more pain in the future puts us into the survival mode. We cannot think of new options. The news media in the USA does an excellent job of covering the most horrific news and sensationalizing it. People are brainwashed to believe in the worst, to expect the worst. This "programs in" fear-beyond-fears. In a brainwashed, fearful state we just react out of all the fear and pain of the past. People in fear, and therefore survival, cannot think clearly. They can be easily manipulated and controlled. When I lived in The Hague, Holland, homicides were purposely not reported. The authorities had realized that reporting adds energy to instigate more homicides by imbalanced individuals. What about the influence of violent computer games on our children?

Whatever we fear, we draw to us. If you have a fear of dogs, it seems as though every dog in the world finds you until you correct your fear of dogs! In a group of 20 guests, for example, our Siamese cat would select the person who was allergic to or didn't like cats and then attempt to sit on his/her lap!

Some examples follow. We could say that all the topics in the other chapters are also based on fear.

FEAR OF ANIMALS

An example of how we block the neurological flow of energy was found in a client who, at the age of three was bitten by a dog and badly frightened. From that time, he had an irrational fear of dogs. He would not visit friends who had dogs. He would cross to the other side of the street if he saw a dog approaching. He lived in constant fear of the next time he would meet a dog. At age 30, he did not remember the initial incident. However, the deep-seated cellular memory was there with the irrational fear. Fear of animals is a common fear I have found and one that is usually easily corrected in one session.

FEAR OF FLYING

One of my clients had a great fear of flying. He understood the reason. When he was eleven, he was put on a plane to meet his father in another city. Upon takeoff, the plane developed mechanical problems. The passengers thought it would crash. They made a safe emergency landing back at the airport of departure. This eleven-year old was not only frightened about the possible crash, but neither parent was there to meet him at the airport nor to help him onto another plane, further adding to his trauma.

As a result, in his adult years he was so terrified of flying he always had to be intoxicated before getting on the plane. He had tried many therapies, including the airline's therapy program, but none worked. Departing from London one Christmas day, there were no liquor stores open. He got to the plane but refused to board. The pilot came out and tried to coax him onto the plane. He explained the situation, so the pilot brought out liquor from the plane. It took 20 minutes to get him intoxicated; then the plane took off. After a 30-minute session with me, he has been able to fly -- alcohol free. We were able to disconnect the fear from that memory. Now it is only a memory without the stress that had been fused into it. White-knuckled-flying-people seem to sit next to me often on my many flights!

~

An American friend had great stress on flying. After my work with him, he had no stress when flying to England. On the way back, he got up to get something out of the overhead compartment and saw a man in back of him giving himself a shot of insulin. He felt very faint. We then had to work on his fear of needles after he returned!

FEAR OF LADDERS/HEIGHTS

In one of my seminars, a student spotted an open spiral staircase in the corner of the theater. She instantly had a deep sinking feeling in her stomach and became very nervous. She was not able to concentrate because those formidable stairs loomed over her! Her fear also extended to bridges. In class, she volunteered for her "fear-of-open-stairs" correction. We went back to the cause, when she was in a park with her father at age two. Her father forced her to climb a steep ladder up to the top of a tower. It was not a problem for her when stairs were enclosed. Open stairways, such as the pull-down stairway into her attic, could not be negotiated.

The body programs in the stress from the original, the first memory of fear. Whether the individual is consciously aware of it in the present or not, the stress remains. After her stress release, she walked over and climbed the open, spiral staircase with ease and pride of accomplishment. We all cheered!

That night she asked her husband to pull down the stairs to their attic. He laughed -- until he watched her bound up the stairs without a problem! I heard from her recently that she is enjoying life much more now that this fear is gone. She traveled over a bridge to Manhattan with no problem and felt completely at ease. She may continue to maintain the memory of that event when she was two, but no longer is she controlled by the stress she formerly had on it.

~

One of my Polish clients had a coordination problem. Each time she moved one hand, the other hand would follow in that movement. She could not disconnect the synchronized movements of the two hands. As a teacher it was very embarrassing to her. She would hide her other hand under her desk while in class when writing or performing similar tasks so the children would not notice.

She had searched for solutions with numerous experts for many years and had given up. We went back to an early age when she was told that she had fallen from a table. After we had made that connection and reactivated the energy system, she was able to isolate the hand movements. I was surprised myself at the quick results. Of course, she was elated! As with most corrections, this one has held over many years.

FEAR OF PUBLIC SPEAKING

Public speaking is one of the greatest fears in the USA today. I can identify closely with this. Speak for 1200 people for one hour? That prospect would leave chills of fear running up and down most people's spines. From where did that fear come? How can we be rid of it? When in university, I would be up all night worrying about giving a five-minute speech in class. My first night in Budapest in 1992, I lectured for 1200 people. It was televised and I had a great time. What was the difference? The fear was gone.

Most of us were not born with the fear of public speaking; we acquired it. This fear is not really a part of us, so we can also remove it just as we would remove a piece of clothing. As tiny babies, we express openly and freely. We coo, laugh, and cry. We don't care who is listening...that is, until someone gives us the message that it is not correct or safe, through comments, body language or punishments!

~

One of my friends, at age nine months, was standing, crying in her crib. Her mother told her in later years that her father came in and spanked her one swat across the backside. She sat down and never really expressed herself freely and openly for the next 50 years. Then, she was introduced to specialized kinesiology. After one session she unleashed all that powerful expression which had been held back for all those years.

~

Deep subconscious programs are planted very early in the brain/body. Each subsequent negative experience creates a deeper degree of fear. How many times in school were we criticized, or even chastised, when we said something "they" considered wrong? Was it the incorrect answer, word, time, or place? This kind of event causes stress hormones to be created that can affect the energy flow. If there is emotional stress when speaking, it can block the normal channels for the speaking mechanisms to work properly. Our thoughts have the power to control our physical and mental actions. Then we are reacting out of the fear and pain of our yesterdays' traumas. Many of us experience "weak legs" and may collapse when we receive shocking news. This is an example of how a negative thought can affect the body.

With specialized kinesiology, we are able to correct the fear of public speaking. I have facilitated hundreds of people in releasing this fear. It usually takes only one session. We are able to access that original memory which was stressful so long ago and then restore the body/brain to its normal neurological flow. When stress enters the picture, it takes three seconds to program a blind spot concerning a specific function. We live with the effects for a lifetime, unless we reprogram our memories.

~

Recently I worked with a very successful international lawyer on her fear of public speaking and composition of her speech. She always felt as though she had lumps in her throat when speaking in public. We also talked about speaking from her heart. This correction process was intended to help her in her legal profession, plus, she was running for an election at the time. This is her email to me days after her session and her subsequent public speech:

"Regarding the speech, it was dynamite! I did not have any lumps in my throat, I spoke clearly and convincingly. Many people came to me after the speech to congratulate me for such an articulate and well thought through speech. Someone even asked whether I wrote it or had it written for me. What a ridiculous question, it was about me and my life, of course I wrote it."

~

I worked with a twelve-year old boy at Camp Artek, at the Black Sea, on stage in front of 400 other children, for his fear of public speaking. At first he turned his back to the audience, he was so shy. After the correction, he took the microphone and sang for five minutes in his native language of Kazakhstan. It was not only a great success for him, but also for the 400 other children witnessing his changes. They could realize their own infinite potential which is inherent in all of us -- when we are cleared of the related stress.

~

When I am demonstrating this correction in a lecture, I must be careful that the newly freed-up speaker does not take over! After the change, I ask them to think about speaking for 20 people, then 200, then 2,000, then 2,000,000! Their muscles test strong on all numbers which means they have no further stress on it.

I ask them how that feels when they think of speaking for so many people. Invariably, they say, it doesn't matter how many people are present. I then tell them I will watch for them on televison!

We can all be public speakers, but sometime in our past, someone told us we couldn't -- and we believed them. Much of our public speaking fear comes from our earliest experiences in school. The fear gets layered over with each negative situation and becomes a very deep pain for us. The good news is that we can correct the stress of public speaking.

Speak for 1,200 people, 12,000, 12,000,000 -- my pleasure! About what would you like me to talk -- and, for how many days?

~

I was about to do a televised show in Bratislava when the hostess asked me if I was nervous. I replied that I was not since I had corrected that fear and did TV shows often. I then asked her if she was nervous. She said that she was fearful and got butterflies in her stomach before every show. I quickly did a session with her with the result that she was completely relaxed on the show. It made for an interesting example for the program! I have been known to stress release the camera-men also!

Not long ago, I gave a two-day seminar for public speaking to a business group in Baltimore. After one and a half days of clearing stress from early childhood on speaking, and also clearing stress on the basic skills, the participants prepared a five-minute speech. The assignment was to introduce themselves to us in a creative way, focusing on a basic theme. These were individuals who, until that moment, had great fear surrounding any kind of presentation to a group of people.

The whole class was in awe at the quality of the content and presentations of their classmates. Since that seminar, I have remained in touch with many of these individuals. They tell me how well they are doing, not just in public speaking, but in other areas of their lives. The effects of one issue can, and usually does ripple out to affect many other areas of one's life in a positive way.

FEAR OF PEOPLE

As a teenager, one of my clients was invited to a religious gathering. There were many people crowded into an undersized meeting room. Suddenly the lights were dimmed and an outer ring of men locked arms in a circle around the gathering. Those inside the circle were essentially barricaded from escaping. There was a clergyman within the circle who was presumably assaulted and stabbed by one of the participants. It was all very real and frightening to my (then) teenage client. Later he learned that it was all staged to test their faith. Fifty years later this event was still so vivid in his mind. The after-effects on certain aspects of his lifetime from this single event have been devastating. His fear of crowds, especially religious or service oriented groups and of being trapped in a situation was a deep, lifetime problem. These fears abated after one session. What happens to young people mentally and emotionally when they go through a hazing at school?

A Polish student had a difficult time with writing. She hated to do it, was poorly coordinated for it and didn't like the way her writing appeared to her. Our research showed the age of cause was one day before her birth. At that time her pregnant mother was living in a village where the German soldiers were approaching from one side and the Russians from the other side to meet in their village for the battle. Can you imagine the added stress with having a baby due at the same time? Many of the same muscles are used in carrying buckets of water as in writing.

We know from our thousands of case studies that the stress of the mother goes into the fetus and can affect any part of the brain/body because the mother and fetus are so closely connected. Our student was very happy with the results of the stress release. Not only did her writing improve immediately, but her emotional stress associated with all aspects of writing was over!

~

Many adults have fear of doctors' offices because of the painful experiences with vaccinations, etc. as a young child. My client was the owner of a building firm. He was very concerned about his high blood-pressure. The pressure was high only when he visited his doctor. Before and after the visit it was normal. His doctor wanted to put him on medication. We were able to surface an event when he was very young when his doctor suddenly came from behind him and gave him a shot. When we got in touch with the base cause of his fear, his blood-pressure returned to normal limits during subsequent visits to his doctor. Blood-pressure medication was not necessary.

FEAR OF AUTHORITY

A new tricycle with a horn can be the gift of a lifetime for a five-year old, that is, if the horn is not silenced against his will! This client's uncle, annoyed by the beeping horn in the household, removed the batteries. The child begged, pleaded and cried, but there was no alternative. It was black and white. The adults, including his mother, were not willing to compromise! They flatly decided that it was going to be that way with no explanation to the child. The child wanted to have the complete toy. Children are by nature perfectionists and they appreciate wholeness. These adults had taken away part of the function of his brand new and much loved tricycle, his Christmas present! The adults didn't care about him; they were not attuned to his sadness. They were cruel! Why wouldn't they let him have his happiness back? The disappointment and sadness of this event was still weighing heavily on this person as he felt those emotions all over again during his session.

As an adult, this experience played out in many avenues of his life in not trusting people, especially "authorities" who could easily take things away from him. People could easily jeopardize his happiness. It also contributed to his very strict black and white thinking. He didn't enjoy Christmas and gift giving or receiving after that. When I heard his story, I finally realized why my daughter has never forgiven us for removing the horn on her toy plastic motorcycle. As parents we must learn to use solutions which do not compromise the relationships with our children's trust.

~

Only a decision is required to change one's mind. How do we reach a decision to change our minds about a conditioned fear for which we may not even recognize the origins? We must go back and address the original cause and clear out the emotion associated with it. Many systems of our world today, especially education, are fear-based. This is an enormous trap for humanity. When we act out of fear, we are not thinking of other options and solutions for problems but are compounding the problems. We spend so much time and energy on feeling and acting out of fear. If you channel that energy to finding and acting on the best solutions to problems then you too can spread your wings and fly!

CHAPTER 2

EMOTIONAL PAIN

What is pain? It is difficult to deal with emotional pain, because you cannot put your finger on a location as you can with a physical pain. Emotional pain may eventually sift down to the body level and become physical pain. Dr. David E. Bresler, former director of UCLA's Pain Control Center, who uses acupuncture, biofeedback and guided imagery when conventional treatment does not work, says, "Pain is a sensation, a perception, an emotion, cognition, a motivation, and energy. I find it difficult, if not impossible to isolate the individual components of pain since it is such a highly integrated, multifaceted phenomenon."

Biofeedback is the major area in which we work in specialized kinesiology. Creative imagery, that is, imagining a better situation, is also a major part of our interaction with clients. In addition to releasing the stress on a memory and balancing the energy flow, we must also visualize a better condition/situation. Every invention is first a thought in the inventor's mind before it becomes a reality. Thus, with our healing, we must also visualize what "better" is, in order to create it! Sometimes, individuals have difficulty imagining how life will be if they are better after they have been ill for so long. When stress from the fear and pain of the past is relieved, and the energy flow is restored, then the body has an excellent chance to rejuvenate.

~

A three and a half-year old stuttered, could not say her initial consonants and mixed up the ends of her words. She was shy and withdrawn.

Through stress testing (biofeedback), I found that the initial cause occurred at age two. At that time, her mother recalled that her father, in a fit of rage, had thrown her and her baby brother down the stairs. I restored energy to the meridians to release this "brain-cell-programmed" stressor. She was immediately able to speak without impediment. She also went over to the stairs and ran up and down them delightedly. Her mother was surprised and said that, since early on, she had been frightened of stairs (and for good reason). The following week, her preschool speech teacher reported that her pronunciation was normal and she didn't stutter. She also became a social butterfly since she could now trust people and feel confident around them. Emotional stress can and does create many kinds of physical blockages.

~

A Polish student (a psychologist) in one of my seminars had seen everything filtered through orange spots from the time that she was a young child. During her volunteer stress release session in class, we went back to age eight. She recalled waking up one morning, looking out the window and seeing all of Warsaw on fire. After releasing the stress on that memory the orange spots were gone for the first time in 60 years. No longer was her beloved city and everything around her being destroyed.

~

At age 80, my mother often emailed me. She was reading books related to my work and telling me the details of the latest book she had read. She was one of the greatest supporters of my work. She would delight in having a session with me.

One time she had an issue with her neck, a pain, and asked for a stress release session. We looked at age ten when she was good at art and winning awards at school. She kept her art materials in a bottom dresser drawer away from her little brother and sister, but her mother would allow both to get into her drawer. She was very clever and changed the drawer pulls to the inside of the lower drawer, but her mother then opened the drawer for the little ones and they made a mess of her materials. She then threw all of her art work and materials away and never did art work again!

When we did the session, even though it was so many decades after the event, she was still so angry about it all. When she could forgive and release, the neck pain vanished. Those siblings and her mother had been a pain in the neck for her! The emotional pain prompted the physical pain which became cumulative over a lifetime. What else had she given up doing that she enjoyed because of others frustrating her?

~

A retired Hungarian dentist attended our first course in Budapest. He had such bad arthritis in his fingers accompanied by pain and numbness. He retired because he could not feel how much pressure he was exerting and would sometimes damage a patient's teeth.

We found the age of cause to be at three years. He was playing in his sandbox with his toys near the Danube River when, suddenly, planes were coming overhead to bomb the city. In their panic, his parents grabbed him while he was using his fingers in play. The parents fear was transferred to him as they rushed off to the bomb shelter.

When we released the fear, energy returned to his fingers and he had mobility and feeling without any further pain in his hands and fingers. The next weekend he came for the next part of the course, pain free. Then we corrected his stress in hearing and vision. He was a happy man! For many years afterward, he sails his boat on the Adriatic Sea with his body functioning well. His negative emotions associated with the previous arthritis pain were also released.

~

The husband of one of The Czech Republic's most famous actresses had recently died from lupus. During one of my seminars that she was attending, she disclosed that she had just been diagnosed with the same disease. I worked with her on the emotional cause and released the stress associated with an earlier traumatic event in her life. At the next seminar she told me she was lupus free. The last time I saw her she was still fine, with no recurrence of lupus.

~

I have conducted many seminars in Hungary for preschool teachers. It is so important to stress release teachers because of their enormous influence on children. It is even more important to work with preschool teachers since the years before six are the most formative time for the child. This is when they develop their self image as well as their beliefs about the world and about people. The teachers in my seminars not only developed a new understanding of how children learn, but also how they become blocked for learning. One teacher had a deep correction on her own anger. At the next seminar she announced to the class that she no longer beat her preschool children, and no longer beat her own child! We were all shocked at the realization that this kind of teacher behavior was still going on, even in Eastern Europe. Now all that behavior has changed for the better for this teacher.

No matter how hard a teacher may attempt to do things differently, that early programming of their own experiences may come through. They may not even be fully aware of what they are saying or doing because they, at that moment, are not thinking of the options for handling a specific situation. They are not in control of what they are saying or doing. They are reacting out of their fears from the past. Their parents and teachers were their models, the people from whom their habitual actions of today were learned. After corrections, they can choose a different way of treating children.

~

I was instructing a group of music teachers in Slovakia. When we checked, they all had stress on music. Most of this went back to when they had teachers themselves who were abusive. For example, one of our teachers gave up singing when her fifth grade teacher said she sounded like a crow! After our changes, their music and lives were much more harmonious.

~

After a lecture in Bratislava, a violinist came to me and asked if I could correct his hand. Because of numbness, he could no longer finger the violin and had to quit his profession playing in the symphony in Vienna. In a few minutes, his hand was perfect!

~

I worked with another very famous musician in Warsaw who had a serious problem with alcohol. After many years, I received an email that he was performing in New York and doing well.

PANIC ATTACKS

Panic attacks are a build up of stress which manifests as "overwhelm" for the individual at a given moment and under certain circumstances. I have had great success working with this problem. Many times panic attacks can be corrected in one session. At times it may require several sessions to resolve the deeply layered root problems. The causes can be many and cumulative.

~

A young lady came to me with a problem of panic attacks. In addition she had two benign tumors on her pituitary. Her doctor did not want to operate. At times she could feel the pressure in her eye (from the tumor pressure on the optic nerve), especially when she was upset emotionally. She used homeopathy and said that it had helped partially.

When she was three, she was running down an incline in her home, fell against a cupboard and split the flesh of her head open. The injury was described to her as "like a rose unfolding". Her parents had warned her not to run there. Her mother had a panic attack at that moment and her brother was crying wildly for her as she was rushed to the hospital to be sutured.

When she and her brother were children, her mother would panic whenever there was a problem. Her family had many tragedies. Her great grandmother died in Auschwitz. With their fear of loss hanging over them, the grandmother and mother were addicted to each other and felt it was an expression of love.

My client and her mother had the same addiction. At age 32, she still talked with her mother two to four times per day. If she did not do as her mother dictated, then her mother felt that her daughter did not love her – and told her so. Her mother was likely to panic if her daughter did not please her. It takes one person to give out the emotional pain and another to accept it. Pain makes us all at least feel something, as negative as it may seem!

In seven years of marriage, my client and her husband had been on only one vacation/event without her mother. My client could not breathe deeply. She said it seemed like someone was sitting on her chest! Guess who!

My client hid her panic attacks from her mother because she did not want to upset her. She felt that she had created her own panic attacks to keep her mother away so she could breathe. When her mother called from her brother's home, upset with the situation there, my client had a sympathetic panic attack in honor of her mother's upsetting time at her brother's home!

Needless to say, we worked on the separation of their energies and guilt concerning her mother. I asked her what she would tell herself as that little three year-old girl. She said she would tell her that she did not have to feel guilty for no longer carrying that package of responsibility for her mother's happiness, a huge burden in her life. She was so relieved and said that she felt a huge weight and pressure off her chest. She could now breathe more easily.

~

This client's husband then made an appointment for her mother to see me the next day. The mother's story is the following: Upon arriving, the mother wanted to work on the same issue as her daughter. It is very helpful when two people are willing to work on a relationship. When asked, the mother did not know why she came to see me. She said it was because her son-in-law told her to come. I asked her what stressed her most in life and she said it was her two children's problems. When I asked what problems, she said it was their jobs and their personal relationships. Her son was in another country and she had many arguments with her daughter.

Before he died her husband told her that she had an unhealthy relationship with her mother. She said she did not want to cling to her children now. She gave an example that when she is in a bad mood and talks to her daughter on the phone, her daughter picks up her bad mood.

Next she told me about her family history. Her mother was paranoid for nearly 30 years and had just passed away two months prior. She was always there for her mother and it took a lot of energy out of her emotionally. Her mother would say things that were irrational although she was normally very bright. Even with six locks on her door, she said that bad people were coming into her apartment and doing nasty things to her. My client's grandmother and grandfather had died at Auschwitz. Her mother was 23 when she was taken there with them, but she had survived.

We had to look at age ten when she moved to Israel. She had to go to school there but did not speak the language so this was extremely stressful. Her mother had wanted to go to Israel, but when she got there she did not like it and wanted to go back to Hungary. Her mother complained continuously. She felt that she should make up to her mother for all her bad experiences and that it was her responsibility to make her mother happy. Her mother expected it. She said her temperament is light, but that her mother sucked all the energy out of her.

When my client was 14, the family moved back to Hungary with many new challenges. There she had to pass a Russian exam after studying for one-half year, where the other children had studied the language for four years. She had heart palpitations then which was scary. She was diagnosed with an under-active thyroid and began medication which she was still taking. As the older sister, she was blamed for all the things her brother did.

When she went to see a friend, her mother was resentful and compared how much time she spent with her and how much time with the friend. In the hospital just before her mother's passing, she told her mother that she did everything for her she could. Her mother replied that she did more than she needed to do.

She could never make her mother truly happy, because her mother was an unhappy person. We are not responsible for another person's choices and happiness. We came into this world alone and we will go out alone. Our choices in life are our responsibility -- and no one else's.

My client had to realize the addictive pattern she had developed with her mother and that this behavioral pattern was now transferred to her relationship with her daughter. They both needed to establish borders and live their own lives. They needed to break this generational pattern so they can each live their lives more fully and be rid of the destructive package passed on to them.

As a vital part of the stress release process, I always ask clients at the end of the session how their lives would be different without the stress. She had to imagine making friends, going on vacations without her daughter and son-in-law and being free of the control issue which bound her to her daughter. Her story is an excellent example of how some generational patterns are passed down: heredity and environment.

She appeared to be transformed at the end of the session and asked if she could see me again, saying that we should have met earlier. Everything has its time. Perhaps she was not ready, earlier, for this release.

EATING DISORDERS

The United States has the highest obesity rates in the world, with 67 per cent of the adults and children over weight, according to "Time" magazine of December 1, 2008. Other nations are rapidly following the American pattern. Fast food and lack of exercise contribute greatly to this trend. The growth of the fast food chains has made high-fat, inexpensive meals readily available. How are the eating habits of children programmed? The tastes that a child develops in childhood are retained into adulthood. They develop a taste for fats and sugar at a very early age, especially in baby food and drinks. A European Union study showed that 95 per cent of the food advertising for children encouraged children to eat foods high in sugar, salt and fat.

What is the cost to individuals and society? Obese people suffer from low self-esteem and emotional pain. Obese American children are dying from heart attacks and other related diseases. Obesity can be the root cause of deaths relative to heart disease and other major causes of death. American health care costs are in the hundreds of billions of dollars annually from obesity. It was estimated that 280,000 Americans die every year because of the results of being overweight.

In addition to exploring the physical reasons for obesity, we also examine the emotional causes: our attitudes and actions with food, including the conditions of anorexia and bulimia. Learn how to take responsibility for your eating habits; it's an inside job! Learn how to behave in front of food! Why do some people diet, exercise, eat very little and still have a weight problem?

~

Now let us look at some emotional causes of eating disorders. The majority of obese clients' biofeedback tests sexual abuse as the cause of their overweight. They say they felt that if they made themselves less attractive, the person abusing them might stop doing so. People also build up physical insulation or protection because they feel so emotionally vulnerable. They may eat to feel fulfilled, because they feel unfulfilled in life. They may over eat because they want to fulfill another's expectations. There often are many levels of stress to remove. What programs are running from your early childhood concerning eating habits? My mother and other family members told me so often how thin I was as a new born and that my fingers looked like bird claws. I have never had a weight problem. If children were told that they were so chubby and cute would they create that in reality for later life?

~

A client had her gallbladder removed. Her doctor told her that she would blow up like a blimp after the operation; she quickly fulfilled his expectation. We released that major stress associated with this client's "programming" received from an "authority" figure. I recall that, when I had my first baby, I had gained more than the doctor thought necessary and he said that I would soon be forty, fat and fertile! I did not meet his weight expectation!

~

One of my student's parents died when she was in her teens and she had to go live with her aunt and her aunt's husband. This uncle watched and commented upon everything she ate so that she would hide to eat. In later life she had so much stress on eating that she wanted to eat in a closet! It was a huge issue and resulted in a great emotional release. Thereafter, she was free to end her fear concerning eating and balance her metabolism.

~

Many years ago a young lady came to me who was anorexic. Her parents had spent $48,000 for one month cure at a well know clinic, with no results. We worked on her relationship with her stepfather at a very young age. She was corrected on that relationship for a specific issue and on the anorexic condition. What is it in life that we can't "chew", that we can't "swallow", that we can't "stomach", that we can't "digest", and that we cannot "eliminate" in our lives? That is where the meridian flow will be interrupted to a specific organ or system and we will likely have a problem there.

Over the years, I have corrected many clients on the emotional cause of eating disorders with excellent results for most. Sometimes it requires more than one session. Some clients do not correct the physical problem, but a least we have corrected the emotional problem behind it and they may need to work further.

ROBBERIES

A client had been robbed many times: three regarding family inheritances, several occurrences of bad advice with securities investments and robbed physically of possessions while on different trips to Europe. We had to go back to age six when he had a prized toy pistol stolen from the front porch of his home by the home-delivery paper boy. He still remembered the name of the paper boy and still called him a low life scum. This situation brought up many issues with which he had to deal, including letting go of the past and of material things, of being careless (thus attracting the robberies), blaming others for his losses, and a money issue that "there is never enough" that caused him to be greedy. He was able to come to terms with past grievances and became more generous in all aspects of his life.

JUDGING OTHERS

Being over-critical was the issue for the session. At age 33, a portion of this man's job was to evaluate others in his business environment. He was always hard on himself and therefore equally hard on others who did less than a perfect job. In grade school, he felt that he was not perfect because he could not excel at sports. He also wanted to get the best grades and to be popular. In his earliest years, he was never allowed to play with other children; therefore, he had no experience with playing basketball, softball, or football.

Because he had been isolated from other children and therefore had few acceptable social skills, the two dreams of excelling in sports and being popular remained just dreams that were not realized. However, he did excel academically without even trying. When invited into an advanced curriculum at one juncture in his elementary school education, he did not choose it because his family (the source of his dysfunction) could see no value in it.

Many realizations came with his stress release session. One is that we are perfect in our own way at a specific point in time. The pain that he had felt throughout his family life and career with his penchant for perfectionism took its toll on him and those around him. After our session, he was able to release some of this criticism of himself and others. He was able to relax and enjoy the diversity within people who do not meet his expectations and most of all to relax when he does not meet his own high standards.

~

Digestive problems have been a major problem and stress around the area of food for a client. He had little respect for obese individuals. He would be concerned about the weight and eating habits of those close to him and weigh himself often, check on others' weight and obsess about how much food others ate. He was openly judgmental about other's weight and eating habits. In checking his family history, I found that his mother and grandfather had the same attitudes. After our session, he recognized the futility of his thinking process. Today, he is a different, happier person regarding this issue.

SUICIDAL

I will now include my story from many years ago, about a young Russian lady who was suicidal. The setting is 1991, Moscow. The Russians have recently been liberated from 70 years of communism. They are told that now they may have freedom, but have no idea what that means. What is freedom without opportunity? The clothing stores are empty. There is no food in the shops. They stand in line for hours in the frigid streets only to find there is nothing left to buy. The Russian ruble continues to be devalued, eventually going from one per dollar to 4,000 per dollar and then much worse. There is an eerie darkness that hangs over the city. February is dark, dank and dismal. The snow, the clothing, the buildings, their lives, all match this. I emerge from America's technicolor world to one of black and white, or more correctly, gray. Many people turn to alcohol to get them through the day. The dream of communism as well as the buildings and the people's lives are perceived by all to have crumbled.

I am invited to the city of Dubna which was closed to the world because of it being the top Scientific Research Center of the former USSR. Before The Wall came down, no one there was allowed contact with the outside world. I am asked to work with their top scientists, whose stress is very high. They appear to be devoid of emotion and so much into their left brain/logical functioning that this state of being has left a great depression in their lives and thinking. It is a new experience for me to see this extreme condition in human life. Their experience and view of the world is very different from mine. It is an education for me, also a pleasure to help these men and women get rid of some of their fear from the past.

As we lumber back to Moscow on an ancient train, there is a call for a doctor. No doctor is available so my interpreter volunteers my services. The young lady in question was about to commit suicide. As I talk with her through my interpreter, she reveals that she had been a professional pianist, but was so emotionally disturbed that she could not pursue her profession any longer. She was divorced with a five-year old daughter. She had to live in the same apartment with her abusive ex-husband because of the lack of living spaces in general. Part of her horror story included having been raped by four men in the back of a taxi. Her co-op leader had told her she should be a prostitute as she was good for nothing else. At the train station in Moscow I work with her a bit more and then I tell her where I would be the next day if she needs more help.

The next day she appears where I am teaching a seminar for a very large group of doctors. I do a session for her. Her goal is to return to her field of music. At the close of the session, she goes to the microphone and tells her life story. The listeners can identify with the tragic story of her life because in many ways it is theirs also. Gracefully, this beautiful young lady moves to the piano on stage and plays the most resounding rendition of classical music; then the finale : "If It Takes Forever". There is not a dry eye in the hall as the significance of a life changed comes to light.

April finds me back in Dubna to speak for an international peace conference for UNESCO, when I am invited to this young musician's new music studio where she performs a concert for me! This young lady touched my life profoundly, taught me a lot about life and love and will always have a special place in my heart, and, I -- in her heart as well.

ROAD RAGE IN A MODEL T

While riding in the car with an older friend, I was puzzled as to why he sometimes cursed other drivers. He would give them the "You stupid idiot look" or mumble under his breath about their driving habits. He was especially critical of female drivers.

At first he didn't want to look at this issue. "It's not my problem, but the other drivers", he would say. When I asked him if it made him feel good when he reacted with this behavior, he replied no. I asked him if he thought it made his "victims" feel good and become better drivers. He again said no. Then I popped the question, "Would you like to be finished with that behavior?" Reluctantly -- he replied yes.

How that ego likes to hold onto those old behavior patterns! We have so much time, energy and emotions invested in them! I asked him next who his model was for this driving behavior. He immediately replied and the mystery was solved. At age six, his Uncle John would often drive with him to the A & W Root Beer stand in his Model T Ford, muttering about inattentive drivers as he went. I am surprised to realize how old road rage is -- Model T's -- horse and buggy days -- perhaps as far back as the chariots!

~

I have been observing driving habits in many countries. While living in Paris and on Sicily, the drivers seemed to be impatient, honking their horns often. On the other hand, in The Hague, if I asked directions, the driver would say "follow me", turn around from his intended destination and escort me clear across town! This happened several times in other towns in Holland. In Warsaw, when a driver sees you coming from a side street, he will slow down and politely allow you to enter before him. What can we learn from their behaviors? When an individual is calm, it is usually reflected in his outer expressed actions.

DEPRESSION

A client was depressed all her life. The root, she said, was that she couldn't feel free. She is an editor. She wanted to write books but couldn't get started. She felt very lonely. She was divorced and her two children had their own lives as adults. She was an only child and never felt close to either parent. She said her parents didn't have the capacity to love.

At age three, she lived in a tiny village where there was no danger, where everyone knew her and she could run freely. The kindergarten and school were together in a large house. She would go to school with the older children and sit with them and pretend to write with a pencil in hand. They called her "little bird", and she liked that. Then, she had to leave all of that behind when the family moved to a bigger village.

She remembered that her mother made a swing for her. It was in the garden surrounded with beautiful plants. She remembers sitting on her mother's lap for the last time; her mother showed her no affection after that event. Later, but still at age three, her mother burned her hand with oil which then blistered. When her daughter touched the blister, it was painful. Her mother scolded her daughter, blaming her for the extra pain she felt. From that point, her mother often verbally abused her, blaming her for everything that went wrong in their home life.

When she started school officially, her mother wanted her to excel, so she always strived to meet her mother's expectations. It was at that time she began to have headaches and stomach aches. Her father was also cruel. Her mother told her bad things about him. However, her mother told her, she (her daughter) had to love him anyway, but she could not. When my client had her own baby, she finally knew what it meant to be a mother and to give love to a child.

We had many issues to resolve. My client left much lighter and happier than she had been one hour earlier. The stress was now gone. She was freed to write her books, free to spread her wings and fly!

CHAPTER 3

PHYSICAL PAIN

A S stated in Chapter Two, emotional pain prompts physical pain and physical pain prompts emotional pain, so it can be a vicious cycle. When we clear the emotional pain from the past, the physical body can heal itself, sometimes instantly. Following is the testimony of an individual who came to me with great pain and many major physical problems at age 73:

"In March, 2006, arthritic-like pain in my feet, ankles and knees was so great that I was not able to stand in the bathroom to brush my teeth or shave unless I first took two over-the-counter pain-alleviating drugs and waited in bed until the drug began to take effect.

I would need to take two more pain-alleviating tablets every four hours during the day in order to walk with some relief while sightseeing, going to lunch, to shop, to and from public transport locations, to whatever normal daily functions I encountered. The level of pain would vary, sometimes requiring that I get out of bed during the night to take more tablets.

It was in that month, March, when I concluded that it was no longer fun to travel internationally, a pastime I had happily undertaken since my retirement ten years earlier. The pain of getting on and off planes, trains and buses, not being able to walk the length and breadth of European cities to enjoy the parks, architecture and other local scenery, caused me to decide to find a retirement home and hang up my passport. I visited several retirement homes and selected one as the most congenial for spending my remaining active years. I decided to make one last three-month trip to my beloved Europe during the summer of 2006 before filing away the passport. I visited my favorite country France, (for the food!), my old neighborhood and workplace in Geneva, Switzerland, and, lastly, a month in my favorite city, Budapest, Hungary.

It was in Budapest that I met Carol Ann Hontz. Upon hearing my story of arthritic pain and of taking twelve doctor-prescribed medications per day, Carol told me that she could help me through her experienced knowledge of specialized kinesiology. I had never before heard of the things she was speaking about and felt a great deal of skepticism. Nevertheless, I told her to go ahead and practice on me if you'd like.

After only forty minutes of the first session with Carol, I no longer felt pain in my feet, ankles or knees. For the first time in many months, I could walk, pain-free and without the dulling, toxic effect that a pain-alleviating drug gives many people.

In subsequent sessions, Carol identified and took away levels of stress that required two different blood pressure medications. Formerly, without these medications, my blood pressure readings would be around 220 over 110. After Carol's work with me, my blood pressure reading is regularly around 120 over 84, without medication! Within the next two months, I stopped taking nine of the twelve medications I'd been taking before my first session with Carol. I continue to take the remaining medications out of personal choice.

Because I wore inferior hearing protection devices while shooting at a skeet and trap range, my hearing was poor. I needed to constantly ask people to repeat themselves during most normal conversations. After one session with Carol, my hearing has improved substantially. It became almost as good as it was prior to my shooting years.

My prostate had enlarged to the point that I needed to take two doctor-prescribed tablets per day in order to urinate somewhat normally. Even so, I still needed to get up 4-5 times per night. After two sessions on this issue with Carol, I no longer take any such medication and my urine flow is almost normal. I usually do not have to get up during the night to urinate.

Three years ago, I was told that I had the beginning stages of glaucoma and that the pressure within the eyeball was at the upper limit. During my most recent eye examination, it was shown that the pressure had fallen to well within a normal, acceptable range with no present risk of glaucoma. This change also occurred after a session with Carol concerning glaucoma.

Carol helped me with many other issues too numerous to mention here. I can truly say that the work she has done with me has relieved physical pain as well as the emotional pain caused by years of stress associated with being raised in an extremely dysfunctional family situation, five years of military service, and forty years of corporate work at a high level of stress that I mostly brought on to myself.

She has also helped me to understand, for the first time in my life, how to love myself and my fellow human beings. She has also helped me to reach a level of inner peace that gives me great comfort and happiness. It is clear to me that all people, especially those just beginning their career, would lead a much happier and more productive life with the knowledge and changes that I have experienced through Carol's sessions with me and with her teachings."

Next, I want to address a few common health problems which, when the related emotional stress is corrected, the body can regenerate itself quickly.

HEADACHES

When we are stressed, various parts of the body/brain can "take the hit". My grandmother had a migraine headache most of her life. I found out that her father was abusive and had hit her on the head when she was a young child.

This is an example of how physical pain can cause emotional pain and emotional pain can cause a physical problem for a lifetime. I know I could have helped my grandmother; however, it was only near the end of her life that I began studying specialized kinesiology.

~

When we address the emotional cause, headaches usually disappear rather quickly. A teacher in Holland had a migraine headache from the time she was a teenager. We looked to age 16 when she was a year ahead in high school. The other girls were a year older and were allowed to wear lipstick, but she was not. We stress released this situation and her migraine headache disappeared immediately.

~

If an individual sustained a concussion earlier in life, we are able to release the stress through a breathing technique. One young man was not doing well at the university; his final exams were coming up. We went to the time when he fell from a tree and sustained a concussion. His entire academic performance improved immensely afterwards.

~

A 27-year old man in Moscow had an excruciating headache for as long as he could remember. He had been a forceps delivery. After we released the stress on the pressure from the forceps delivery, he had no headaches for the first time in his life.

KNEE PROBLEMS

One of my neighbors had a severe problem with her knee and could hardly walk. She had to cancel her travel plans and could not even carry her groceries from the store.

The emotion associated with knees is often fear of loss. In 1944, when this woman was four, her mother was taken to a concentration camp and never heard from again. After one session, she was able and eager to travel once more and cancelled the surgery. Years later, her knee is still fine.

Recently she had a back and ankle problem which was corrected after eliminating stress with earlier male relationships. Her father had raised her and he was very controlling. We spent a few additional sessions on her stress with men.

BACKACHES

If we become emotionally stressed, our muscles can tighten up on one side more than the other and pull our vertebrae out of alignment. This can result in many problems that can become chronic. As an example, we may have stress with our mother-in-law. She phones us and says something very upsetting. All those muscles on the left side of the body may tighten. We go to the doctor for pain killers or to the massage therapist or chiropractor for an adjustment and we feel better for awhile. The next time she phones the same thing happens. She comes to dinner and that is the limit! You are flat on your back. Until you solve the problems with your mother-in-law, defining your borders with direct, open, honest communication, you're stuck!

~

At my grandmother's funeral, three of my relatives had such severe back problems that they could hardly walk to attend the funeral. I was able to work with two of them.

With one relative, I went back 50 years earlier -- to age 14. She and her best friend were the most popular, intelligent and beautiful girls in their class. They were usually competing for the highest grades. Her friend consistently had at least one-half point higher on her exams than she. After we released the emotion of resentment, her back was perfect and is still good 18 years later.

With the other relative, we went back to age 19 where he was in the military, took a test and got an outstanding score for a promotion. The only problem was that there was no position open. This had been a pattern of disappointing events in his life. After the session, his back was fine. Later he was unable to pick up tools with his right hand. What didn't he want to "grasp" in life?

After the "release" that came from my work with him, his hand was completely flexible. It is interesting to work with family and friends because I can follow their progress over the ensuing years.

~

Several years ago, a gentleman literally crawled into my office with severe back pain. He lay on the floor writhing in pain. After the session he walked out feeling great! I never saw him again! This is a regular occurrence in my work. One session, so often, is all that is needed.

~

A younger brother often caused jealousy for this next client. He and his mother were close and he always tried to have her to himself.

When we researched the emotional cause of his backache, we came to age five where he and his brother each had a tonsillectomy on the same day. He remembered the strong light and the sponge in front of his face and the white light when he awoke.

He had to share his mother's attention with his younger brother in the hospital and at home. After we got in touch with that jealousy and anger in our session, he experienced no more serious backache.

NECK ACHES

During one of my group lectures at a health fair, a young gentleman tried to re-balance his head by moving his head repeatedly forward and his chin sharply up. This made a loud clicking sound from his neck vertebrae. After the lecture he asked for an appointment to see me privately.

He had visited different kinds of specialists over a ten-year period, to no avail. We traced the problem to age nine when he was beaten up by an older boy. We got in touch with the emotions that had been buried since then.

Since forgiveness is a necessary part of the healing process, he had to forgive that boy. Immediately his neck and spine straightened and he no longer moved his head to find balance. His partner was delighted. She said that loud clicking was the last thing she heard at night and the first thing that awakened her in the morning. One session with me resolved this physical problem that many earlier years of treatment did not help -- and helped his relationship immensely!

SKIN PROBLEMS

Spots had started to appear on the face of a client -- red, painful and oozing. The dermatologist told her it was a physical problem, but my client refused medication.

Skin is the border in your physical body. It is highly symbolic of where and how you keep your personal borders. Borders are a matter of stating who you are and what your laws are. Keeping your borders (as well as respecting the borders of others) is vital to well-being.

This client's elderly parents were very ill. Her father insisted that she and her husband move into their tiny apartment. I had worked with the parents and had seen the apartment which consisted of a tiny kitchen, a combined living room/bedroom and another tiny room and bathroom.

This daughter was always a "good girl" and did everything her parents wanted. We looked at age ten when her mother wanted to protect her from everything. She kept her in the apartment and would not let her go out to play with other children. Her mother said her daughter was not healthy, thus she could do very little. She was not allowed to confront her parents -- they knew everything! She was absent from school so much that she had to repeat a grade even though she was very bright. She was taught to comply and to give up her choices.

Her mother's major expression of love was fear. Now with her father's insistence to move in with them, she developed spots on her face. We released her from her "bondage". She was able to tell her father no, and not feel guilty. On the way home from her session the pain was gone, the discharge from her lesions stopped. The next morning the spots were gone! They have not returned. She, finally at age 50, took charge of her life.

~

Another client had a major problem with hives. We worked at age eleven where she had a very big issue with her father. Again it was a problem with borders. The hives first disappeared, but then returned, so we worked on a deeper level. They are now gone permanently it would seem.

~

A professional man had very bad acne as a teenager which left him with deep scars on his face. We worked on the borders with his parents. He still had a major issue with them as an adult. I worked with him on a Monday. By Friday, his face was nearly cleared of the scars. He looks like a totally different person. What a boost to his self esteem.

The following are his words about the scars:

"In my childhood, from about 13 years old, my face was full of acne. This problem was very disturbing and I tried to solve this for myself; I rubbed and gouged my skin. Unfortunately this had a bad result; my face became scarred. After hearing my partner's success with specialized kinesiology, I met Carol and decided to try a session with her. After working on my problems, my face became much better. My skin looked tighter and smoother. I was very happy and very impressed!"

Recently, his parents did not approve of his fiancée. Now she is his wife. He has broken the chains that bound him to his parents. How wonderful it is that they have the knowledge to parent in a different way than they were parented. Note: The emotional scars are also healed.

EXHAUSTION

One of my clients was concerned that she was procrastinating. She always felt so tired and so overwhelmed, she could not do her paper work or clear her office. Her husband had had a stroke. She chose to care for him while continuing her medical practice. He wanted to watch television until midnight so she stayed up to get him ready and help him to bed. Then she got up at six a.m. to walk the dog.

We had to go to age eight when she was also overwhelmed. At this time, she was very caring and trusting. A strange man took her from the street to a nearby sweet shop and bought her a pastry. They stopped on the street before her home and he opened his coat and exposed himself. She never told anyone about this incident. It bothered her very much. We successfully released the stress of that episode.

As a separate issue at age eight, her mother was hysterical and would throw herself on the floor in a fit or begin to jump out the window. Her father was always there to rescue her mother.

Her parents moved with her to a new apartment that year. To add to all this stress, she wanted to buy a doll, but her parents refused. She decided to play with a coin. Her aunt told her that if she swallowed it she would die. It was already in her mouth and the shock of that news caused her to gulp and swallow the coin! The fear stayed with her while the family went on a holiday. They were so happy there, but she knew she was about to die! Because she had been told that her opinions and feelings did not matter, she said nothing. Her lifetime was about obeying and taking care of others.

After our work together, she realized that it is time to take care of her life. She must tell her husband that the television goes off at ten p.m. because she must get her sleep to be able to function properly. We worked on many aspects of her problems to get her focused on her priorities, mainly on communicating and caring for herself.

She left my office feeling a great release with the following message for my book:

"When I met specialized kinesiology, I was in a crisis. I felt guilty because as a physician I could not save my mother. After the session I realized that I had to realized that I must consider myself important if I am to be able to help others."

She is one of our graduates who is using specialized kinesiology in her work as a medical doctor.

BURPING

After surgery, a client began burping and it became a constant, ongoing problem. Her doctor told her she would have to learn to live with it. We worked on her anger at a certain age, restored the energy to the hiatal tendency area and immediately the burping stopped. Ten years later there is still no problem with it.

~

Another client was burping and belching to excess all of his life. We found the cause of it at age two where he learned that, in his family, it seemed to be the thing to do. He said they must have believed it was a part of the digestive process. In reality, they probably picked it up the same way as he, as small children who want to imitate their caregivers. Now he gets through the day with few extra sound effects!

ACCIDENTS

Did you ever have the same type of accident repeat itself? From our work, we realize that if you have certain muscles engaged (a muscle circuit) and have trauma at that time, that muscle combination will remember that stressful situation. Then when you are in a similar situation with that muscle circuit engaged again (same position), your body will remember the trauma and the muscles will go weak and repeat that accident.

A relative fell down the stairs several times. Finally, after she broke her ankle, it was time to seriously address the problem. We found and released the painful memory that affected that muscle group while on the stairs. She has not fallen down the stairs since.

~

A gentleman in Moscow had been in a car accident ten years earlier, had his leg broken in three places and was hospitalized for two years. Although the wounds had healed nicely, he could not work or do much because of constant pain. There appeared to be no reason for this pain. When we took him back to seconds before the accident, he realized that if he had made another choice, he would have avoided the accident. After he forgave himself for that decision, the pain of ten years was gone.

~

While living in The Netherlands, we became avid bicycle riders. While cycling on the bike path with my family, there was a man coming toward me in the middle of the path. I froze. I could not ring the bell. I could not turn the wheel. Crash! Off the bike I went. Later I was vacationing in Holland and this time went bike riding with some friends. One friend stopped suddenly in front of me, but I could not apply my brakes or do anything to avoid running into her.

By this time I had begun studying specialized kinesiology and knew what I had to do to avoid further accidents. The memory flooded back. My oldest sister liked to do lots of tricks with her little sister -- me!

When I was six, I got my brand new, big, two-wheel bike for Christmas. This same sister thought it would be in my best interest if I learned to ride quickly. My sister put me on the bike and pushed me down a long hill in front of our home. Soon the wheels were spinning horizontally and I was lying on the road. Not only did I experience this initially, but our friend had it on film, so we got to see it replayed many times! I have forgiven my sister for all those fancy stunts she did with me and we are the best of friends. My middle sister who felt the brunt of our older sister's creative sisterhood is merciless in reminding her at every opportunity of the "games" she played with us as the older sister! I was able to stress release myself on that memory and have not had a similar accident since.

~

The following is a few words from a friend:

"Carol Ann Hontz has been a dear friend, neighbor and a facilitator of my health for over 20 years. It seems like every time I have a major problem, she calls or shows up in my life!

My physical problems seem to center around my hands, legs, joints, and back. One specific time that Carol showed up was after I had a car accident and my hand was not functioning properly. Carol guided me to understand that on some level we plan our 'accidents' by what we want to avoid, have to learn, or perhaps just to schedule some time-out which we feel we cannot get in any other way. After stress testing, we found out exactly when I programmed in that behavioral pattern. Then we were able to release the stress on that memory. I could immediately feel oneness with my body and to reconnect with my hands. The energy returned, giving me full mobility in my hands again.

Another time Carol showed up was just after I caught my heel in the hem of my pant leg and took a bad spill. I could not walk. We worked on the past emotional stress relating again to why I had punished myself with this accident. In minutes, I walked perfectly!

My sessions with Carol over the years have been so numerous and the results so profound. Europe, Savannah or New Jersey -- we always seem to meet at the right time."

~

Friends from Dubna, Russia came to see me in Moscow. The husband had broken his hand playing football with his child. During his session he said that he was actually glad that he broke his hand. His job and family responsibilities were overwhelming him. Finally he had some time to rest! His wife was sitting there observing the whole thing and she said, "Well, I need a 'break', too!" I worked with her also and afterwards she could understand that there are easier ways to get a rest. It is called planning, scheduling relaxation and vacations into your life. They are able to do that now.

~

A gentleman wrote me the following message:

"I was hit in my car by a drunk driver seven years ago at two o'clock in the morning. After the accident, I was diagnosed with Traumatic Brain Injury. I don't know exactly what happened in my car, but I had significant swelling on the back of my head, especially on the right side behind the right ear. I had lots of back pain for several months in my mid-back. My car was hit toward the rear on the passenger side, and spun around. The driver who hit me was driving at least 50 mph.

My symptoms: double vision, mood swings, significant loss of short term memory, mental fatigue, easily over-stimulated mentally, could not talk to someone if the TV or radio was on as it was too distracting and confusing -- also extreme difficulty with concentration, attention, executive function, processing information. I saw things but didn't "see" them. There are more symptoms but I can't remember them.

I had some gradual improvement, especially the last two years. There was still some mental fatigue, some short term memory problems, but much less. I could go much longer without breaks -- still some perception issues, but less. I have had great success with some products.

I went to a family event last weekend -- flew there on Saturday morning, flew back Sunday night. Since returning, I am having a lot more mental fatigue and perceptual problems than I have had for a while. On Monday, I had difficulty waking up mentally until about four p.m. Today, Tuesday, I had much the same. Waking up mentally is meaning that I feel OK from the neck down, but small mental tasks are very fatiguing, feels like a 'pulled thinking muscle'. Now it is later in the afternoon and I am feeling somewhat better. This was the pattern from yesterday as well. My brain feels like it wants to go to sleep. Also, I am traveling on Thursday to California and need to be in tip-top shape. I am looking forward to your help."

Later, after I worked with him, he said:

"Now, I am doing great and your session with me was most helpful. I was undergoing some severe mental fatigue at the time I saw you. Mental fatigue is typical since I am a recovering TBI (traumatic brain injury) survivor. But, I had been having severe mental fatigue, almost to the point of not being able to pick my head up and get out of bed. After you worked on me, I noticed that my energy was returning (thanks to you). Since our session a couple of weeks ago, I have noticed increased energy, as well as a dramatic decrease in cognitive fatigue. Thank you so much, Carol."

This was my reply to that email:

"Wonderful to hear your good news and we've just begun! It would be positive if you no longer label yourself as a 'traumatic brain injury survivor', but use positive healing energy in thinking of yourself as a healthy, happy human being and all those other fabulous adjectives which you are! As Henry Ford said, 'If you think you can…or think you can't do a thing, either way you are right'!"

~

One of our students came hobbling into our Holiday-Stress-Free Seminar with his foot in a removable cast. He had fallen in his rush to get the Christmas shopping done. He had a lot of pain and the doctor told him he could not put any pressure on his foot for six weeks.

While the other students were working, I invited him to work with me. We researched age three but also had to look at age two when his family took him to the train to get his rocking horse and other Christmas gifts. It was then he learned that Christmas presents arrive on trains (not from Santa?).

Being the thoughtful, adventurous and creative child that he was at age three, he decided that he would go to the train and get all the gifts for the family. However, he was caught by his grandparents toddling down the street on his way to meet the train and was punished.

He learned that Christmas was not much fun and especially on the way to shop for gifts! He didn't enjoy Christmas much after that. As soon as we released the emotional stress, he took off his cast and walked pain free. He never put the cast back on. I don't know what he told his doctor!

~

It is interesting to watch many of our families as the children mature. The following story is from a family where the parents and two daughters were my graduates. (I could write a book on this family alone!) A call came from the hospital from dad to please come to stress release his daughter. She had fallen from her horse and had damaged her kidney. The doctor wanted to operate to discover what was causing the bleeding. When I arrived she was pale, crying from the pain and terrified. After 20 minutes she was laughing, free of pain and went home the next day. She has had no problems since then and it has been several years.

OPERATIONS (SURGERY)

If someone comes to me and asks if they should have an operation, I simply tell them that we can test only to see how much stress they have on surgery. They can then correct the reason for the stress about surgery, so they can be at choice and make a clear decision themselves. I highly recommend sessions before and after surgery, first to get rid of stress, then so the individual can heal as quickly as possible.

~

A neighbor was about to be operated on for an aneurysm and was so panicked about having the anesthetic and going to sleep. We went back to age three. It was a very stressful time in the family as they were all huddled around the radio to hear about the assassination of the head of Hungary, Imre Nagy, the father of her mother's friend.

She remembered being in a tiny bed when her grandmother told her that if she didn't keep her arms and legs covered with the blanket, someone would come and cut them off! She did not want to go to sleep after that. Whenever she went to the market and saw the animal parts hanging there, she panicked. After her session, she sailed through the operation, free of that stress, and recovered quickly.

~

An individual was about to have a back operation. I worked with him before and just after his surgery. In a few days he was walking three miles, having recovered very quickly.

~

My sister had surgery to clear out the scar tissue from a previous operation. Mother called to inform me that after a week my sister was getting weaker and weaker. They were worried about her. She was not eating at all, having no appetite. I immediately drove the three hours from New Jersey to central Pennsylvania to check on her. I found her extremely weak and tired.

We went back to age 24 when her colleague would take long breaks. My sister would have to do her colleague's work, a step that was required before she could continue on with her own work. However, this caused her to get behind in her own work. She did not think that was fair. She did not communicate with her colleague about this. When we go to the past we also relate it to a present-time challenge/problem and ask how your life would be different if we no longer have this problem. What was unfair in her life now that she was not communicating about in her present job?

Her session was very long and at the close of it, she jumped out of the chair, bounced out to the kitchen and exclaimed, "I'm starved! Would you like a cup of tea?" Her recovery was so fast that we were all astonished. The next week she was working in her fabulous flower gardens.

~

One of my seminar graduate's husband was in the hospital about to have an operation for kidney stones. He was in such pain the evening before the scheduled operation that he begged his wife to do a stress release session with him. She did and the pain disappeared. The next morning he told the doctors not to operate because he felt fine, but they insisted. They found no stones.

After leaving the hospital, he resigned from his successful business, and attended all of my seminars (to get his facilitator's certification to teach and see clients). Now he and his wife are doing this work full time. They are extremely successful in their teaching of specialized kinesiology and in their work with clients. They also learned the principle reason I do this work -- the joy and happiness that comes from helping other people to help themselves get well!

~

Another student had great pain from kidney stones during class. We did a session and soon she came back from the restroom with two tiny stones in her hand! Correct the emotions and the body will follow with healing!

~

A client came to me with Lyme's Disease which affected so many areas of her life. She had not heard well in her right ear after having scarlet fever at age six. We researched age ten when she said she had a gruesome year in school. She hated her teacher and another classmate. A brief time after her correction, I received the following email from her:

"I came to see Carol Ann for lingering symptoms of Lyme's Disease. I was feeling very run down and had aches and pains in my body and felt like I had a fever all the time. It's been 2 months since Carol Ann worked with me and I haven't had any symptoms since that time. I had blood tests taken after my meeting with her, and everything came back negative. I'm very grateful for her treatment." -- Testimonial of "S".

CHAPTER 4

RELATIONSHIPS

As Veronica A. Shoffstall states in "After Awhile":

After a while you learn the subtle difference
Between holding a hand and chaining a soul,
And you learn that love doesn't mean leaning
And company doesn't mean security,
And you begin to learn that kisses aren't contracts
And presents aren't promises,
And you begin to accept your defeats
With your head up and your eyes open
With the grace of a woman, not the grief of a child,
And you learn to build all your roads on today,
Because tomorrow's ground is too uncertain for plans,
And futures have a way of falling down in mid-flight.
After a while you learn
That even sunshine burns if you get too much.
You plant your own garden and decorate your own soul,
Instead of waiting for someone to bring you flowers.
And you learn that you really can endure...
That you really are strong,
And you really have worth.
And you learn and learn...
With every goodbye you learn.

HOW many relationships chain a soul? Husband/wife, parent/child, teacher/student? How does your life register on this? If there is a life error of humans, could it be that of chaining a soul? Or an even greater life error of allowing your soul to be chained? How many kisses and presents are taken as contracts? "I am giving you this gift and expect something in return." Oh no, we may not state it verbally, that's too risky. But that is sometimes the intention in some relationships.

Relationships: it is said to be the number one stressor of our times. How are your primary relationships? What about those relationships with your colleagues, your boss, your employees, your parents, your children, your mother-in-law, your friends, your neighbors? Are we into separation and no-choice in those relationships, repeating the same behavioral patterns of control or being controlled for a lifetime?

Can we break those self-destructive patterns that are based on our fear and pain from the past? Through stress release, we are able to break down the limitations that block us in developing healthy relationships. Through awareness we are able to create the kinds of relationships we desire. Those that are filled with love, understanding, compassion and peace.

However, we must keep in mind the most important relationship is with ourselves. With acceptance of self we gain the high esteem that is necessary in the development of our infinite potential. That is the theme of specialized kinesiology (and, of Montessori Education, another topic near and dear to my heart). Again consider our relationships with parents, siblings, friends, partners of all kinds. Even though we have released much of this stress, we must make a conscious choice to behave differently in a given situation in that specific relationship.

~

My young friend's husband left her. She had given up her career to support him and to care for their son for seven years. She was totally distraught and didn't have purpose in her life when he left her. We did a demonstration in class with a future progression. After releasing the stress from an earlier time, she projected her thoughts into the future where she imagined a different scene, one of being back at her career, of playing in the park with her son in the snow. That night her husband called (after three months of being away) stating to her that he had problems with his back, and other complaints. She replied to him: "I have my own life now; I can't be concerned with your problems."

My student took back her power and got rid of her chains on her soul so she could realize the power within herself. Then she was desirable again. Six months later I was back in Moscow and guess who was in my class? Her husband and seven-year old son! I was able to help her husband also to deal with life in a more positive way.

~

When we have issues with another person, we are burdened with the negative energy of that relationship, so we need to work through it. A retired gentleman had a severe pain in his shoulder and could no longer play the piano, could no longer play tennis well, nor could he enjoy painting on his canvasses. He said that he had no stress now that he was retired.

We found the age of cause at 33 where he had major problems with his boss of that time. A similar scenario was repeated just before his retirement six months ago!

We released the stress in that memory which had lodged finally in his shoulder as resentment. He came to the realization that his bosses did the best they could at the time, given their belief systems and experience of life. He could then let go of that resentment towards them.

Now his only job is to enjoy his retirement and paint another wonderful watercolor for me! We have plans to resume our piano/singing get-togethers, now that his shoulder is perfect.

~

His wife had great pain with her sciatica. Researching the cause we went to age 13 where at camp she had to go on a night walk into the forest. She was very afraid. The body holds our emotional punishment.

We had to do a follow-up session at age eight when she went to her first funeral and did not understand any of the process of dying and death. When we released that, her sciatica pain diminished and soon disappeared.

~

Who is chaining your soul? Whose soul are you chaining? Any person over whom you assume authority or anyone you allow to assume authority over you is a soul-chaining situation. If you're forty and still living at home, dependent on your parents, that can be chains! It may not be advantageous for either you or them. Your dependence on your parents may have blocked independence for all three of you.

How much do you depend upon others for your happiness? Those are chains. How responsible do you feel for another person's happiness? That's a chain. Each individual is responsible for his/her own happiness or unhappiness.

~

Is the government chaining us? There was an interesting photo in Time Magazine with the Parliament Building burning in Moscow (1990s) with a woman in front asking, "Who's in charge of my life now?" Those are chains. Who is in charge of your life?

The master/slave concept goes back thousands of years. Isn't it time we broke the chains that bind and take back our power and take control of our life? Then we can realize what the best choice is for all and live in peace, love and harmony.

~

Another woman's husband had left her five years earlier for a younger woman. She could no longer focus on her job as head of a university and spent her time re-living the past.

After a few minutes of working with me during a private session and talking about the situation and releasing it, she joked, "What husband?" When she was rid of the pain of that past separation, she could be free to have her energy back, to focus on her work and to create a space in her life for a new relationship.

~

What about teacher/student relationships? I don't have to remind most of you of the stories about the experiences you may have had in school when you were a student! Most of us have deep emotional scars from our educational experiences. Those are chains. How many children enjoy their teachers and school so much that they can't wait to go to school each day?

~

A client often had a blood pressure reading over 200. Her doctor could find no physical cause for it. On researching we found the age of cause to be eight years when she got a new teacher in school who did not like her. The teacher had the children wash their hands. Then she said that this little girl did not get her nails clean, held her hands up to show the class and hit her nails with a ruler.

My client at age 50 said she had thought about that event so many times in her life with such shame. She felt great relief after her session. Teachers spend so much time with our children and have such a profound impression on them. It is so important that our teachers get rid of their own fear, anger and pain so they do not reflect it in the classroom.

~

From fifth to eighth grade, I had such a fear of my math and geography teacher that it took me years to get over it. Fortunately, my teacher for the other subjects was fine and I managed well in those years.

~

So, how did we get into bondage? It took a lot of work, heartache, pain and misery. There we are, still wallowing in it. Aren't you tired of it? How did we get into that deep pit? How can we get out? How can we stay out?

How many adults have fear of their parents even though they are parents themselves now? Those are chains, chains which can go on for generations, linking us to self-destructive relationships. How many parents have control issues with their grown children?

~

A client of many years came to me with a "heart pain" which he had had for three months. The doctor could find no cause. Knowing the family well, I asked who was breaking his heart. He replied, "My 20-year old daughter, who will not speak to me. I don't even know where she is." We spoke of their relationship and his need to control her -- which was not working! We discussed that he had to focus on his own life and allow his daughter to focus on hers. Immediately his heart pain was gone and for many years thus far.

~

The first realization we need to make is that we are our best friend or our worst enemy. Whatever is going on within those relationships "out there" is merely a reflection of our self-acceptance or rejection. We can blame all those people out there for our problems, but we will never get better in terms of relationships until we take a good hard look into the mirror! Communication with other people is very important but communication with ourselves is the most important!

COMMUNICATION

One of my foreign friends asked a colleague if he worked on Excel. His colleague replied that, yes, he usually wore XL (extra large). This conversation continued for several minutes until my friend's wife informed them that they were obviously talking about two different things!

How often do we ramble on, not listening to the other person? We assume that we are talking about the same thing and that we have the same understanding. One of the greatest stressors in today's world is the lack of communication, miscommunication, or the direct misleading of another for manipulation and selfish personal gain.

One definition: to communicate is to transmit information, thought or feeling so that it is satisfactorily received or understood.

Beyond that definition, it is important to clear out our stress on a given issue first. Then we may be clear on how we feel and what we want in a given situation. If we are coming to an issue with great fear and anger, we may not see the situation with an open mind. It is OK to express fear and anger, but holding onto it is the danger. Through stress release, we are able to clear issues so we can be more objective.

LISTENING

Listening is a major component of effective communication. I sometimes have my seminar's adult students pair up. One of them talks for five solid minutes while their partner does nothing but listen silently -- no nodding, no comments of any kind! Most listeners of these pairings have difficulty with the assignment, and agree that it is a great challenge.

We must remember that we have ears as well as mouths! Our job is to hear accurately and to comprehend what has been said. To clarify what the person has said, it is good to restate it and ask if that is what s/he meant. This fosters understanding for both persons. We need to learn to listen without judgment, and to understand the feelings behind the message.

~

A client wanted to work on his impatience. We went back to age 40 when he wanted his wife to get a job to help with household expenses. He was forceful and demanding to which she reacted negatively. He would them stomp off in anger and sulk in a corner reading a book and spend days in silence.

After releasing the stress, we talked about how he could break this pattern, which continued on in his later years. He could tell others, first, how he feels in a given situation; next, what he wants and finally, what he is willing to do in that situation to correct it. He also needed to learn to listen to others' view points and consider their feelings. Retreating from social contact had become a deep pattern in his life. It ruled his feelings toward others and he chose to be alone most of his life, never developing any close relationships. He is now a happier, more peaceful person.

TELLING THE TRUTH

In our classes, we analyze what percentage of the time we are lying. How often do we tell the truth about how we feel about a situation, person, place or thing in the moment that we have the feeling? Why don't we?

We do not want to appear less than perfect in the eyes of others. Therefore, we often tell them what we think they want to hear. We may be afraid of offending them or perhaps we doubt that our feelings are correct or appropriate. When we are not honest in the moment, it sets us up for larger problems in the future.

We must communicate effectively and honestly. Otherwise, it can cause major problems in the home, the office, among nations, and, most importantly, within ourselves. When someone is not willing to express openly, they isolate themselves. Many people have been told how they should feel by their parents, teachers and others for so long, that they have a problem sorting out what are their own and what are another's beliefs. If we are not clear with our own feelings, how can we communicate with others?

COMMUNICATING OUR VIEWPOINT AND ACCEPTING OTHERS' VIEWPOINTS

It is important in any relationship that the parties express their viewpoints and feelings directly. There are as many different viewpoints on a subject as there are people involved. If we are standing on our planet, our perception of the earth is very different from someone in an airplane or from someone in a rocket ship orbiting the earth or for someone deep within a coal mine. We all come from a different background, genetic code, and life experience, so our views are naturally different. We may choose to honor, respect and accept another's viewpoints, even though they are different from ours. Being open is the way to begin communication, which will lead to feeling more comfortable, and to feeling empathy and oneness.

When we automatically agree with others without examining our own feelings and expressing them, we lose our identity and become powerless. When our views are in direct opposition, we can air them and work together through the various points toward a strong bond with understanding.

It is advisable to listen to a wide variety of viewpoints and feelings to get a larger picture, a worldview, and then we can reach solutions and cooperate harmoniously. I was told a story of a mother who had one orange and two children, so she cut the orange in two and gave them each a half. One child said, "I wanted only the peel," while the other said, "I wanted only the juice." If all three had communicated, they all could have had exactly what each wanted.

Sometimes we may think that we have complete agreement, when later we find that there are points of disagreement. This is where contracts are helpful when they are very clear and when people uphold them.

When we have clear, direct, open, honest communication, it leads to a smooth decision-making process. What does each person want and how can we reach a decision where everyone wins in that situation?

If in a family, each person is respected and listened to with direct, honest, open communication, it will be a happy family. Visualize a government where all parties are treated with respect and dignity, where differing viewpoints are considered, coming to a mutually beneficial agreement for all. This government is serving its people well. Imagine a world where everyone's views are honored and respected and the people are all focused on finding solutions for the highest and greatest good. In this world everyone wins and there is peace and love on earth. Isn't that the goal we each all long for? It is up to <u>you</u> to make that happen! Communicate!

Since relationships are one of the greatest sources of stress in our modern world, we must take a fresh approach to the reasons we are in relationships. What do we have to do and learn within these circumstances? When we look deeply into the root causes within ourselves we can understand the negative responses and actions we manifest. With clarity and with being "at choice" we can then select another constructive response and action when problems and challenges confront us. Parent/child, student/teacher and primary relationships are our major focus in life! The most important relationship is with ourselves.

CHILD/PARENT RELATIONSHIPS - PRENATAL

The most lasting, closest, and most impressionable relationship, second only to that with ourselves, is that of a child with his parents. We come into this life with a set of blueprints for constructing our lives. Some of us have red hair, blue eyes, are tall. These traits are a given by our genetic encoding, passed down from our parents. From them, we have not only our genetic encoding, but also we take on our parents' belief systems about the world and ourselves. Thus, hereditary and environmental factors are the stage of life which they provide for us. These become the backdrop with which we construct our lives. If the genes are healthy and strong and the environment secure, happy, accepting, loving, and all our basic emotional, mental and physical needs met, then we have a great start for our lives.

It is a universal given that we have some kind of stress with our parents, no matter how ideal that relationship may have been. There had to have been times when there were clashes in beliefs, values, or "something". Even if those relationships seem to be good today, there is usually some stress remaining.

What if you could take yourself back to the womb world when you decided on some level that you would enter this lifetime? What if that developing embryo had a consciousness and could understand what was happening to his parents and the world into which s/he would soon be born? Research tells us that not only do the nutrition and drugs the mother-to-be takes affect the fetus, but also the emotions of the parents and particularly those of the mother. The physical connection of the mother and fetus are direct. A mother's stress is often transmitted to the fetus.

~

I worked with an eight year-old who had trouble learning in school. His eyes had dilated pupils which is viewed as a stress affect; it could result in adrenal overwhelm. We had to go back to the origin of the stress at 13 days before his birth. His mother said that it was the moment when her husband left her. After the release session, the child was so excited, he could see on either side (peripheral vision). He said that before his session with me he could see only just straight ahead. Little wonder that he had difficulty in reading, writing and all areas that required balanced vision. The next morning his mother called and told us that his pupils were no longer dilated. What a difference one stress release session can make in a child's life!

~

Another example of prenatal stress was with a three and a half year-old in Moscow who couldn't walk. The doctors had said she would never walk, but they didn't know why. I worked with her on prenatal stress at three months, when her mother bought an apartment. Because of fraud by the seller, she did not receive it nor was her money returned. Her stress hormones went through to the fetus. After the session the little girl got stronger each day and was walking perfectly in three months. On my next trip to Moscow, she returned to me and wanted to release blocks on becoming a ballerina since many of the little Russian girls love to dance. A month later, I called my manager there and she said the little girl was dancing beautifully. What a metamorphosis this was, literally, in the truest sense of the process!

CHILD/PARENT
RELATIONSHIPS – BIRTH

In this section I will not only talk about relationships but also the birth process itself.

Dr. Leboyer in his book, "Birth without Violence" gives us an excellent model for the birthing of babies when there are no other complications with the mother. He instructs the mother to be in a quiet, warm, natural environment without rough handling, without drugs, loud noises, bright lights. Then the newborn is put immediately on the mother's breast for the warmth and love, hearing her heartbeat and bonding with her. Immediate nursing gives the child antibodies in that first milk.

From observing how cats gave birth, Dr. Lamaze established a very well known breathing method for birthing children. It is a natural, stress free approach involving the participation of the father or other family members. We experienced this in the birth of our first daughter many years ago.

My husband carried her back from the delivery room, and we called our relatives to tell them the news and celebrated that beautiful new little life. If emotional stress and fear is released from the belief systems surrounding the birth process, then most times, it can be a calm, joyous experience.

In some primitive societies the women pause in their work, have the baby, put the baby in a sling on their backs and go right on working. They have not been programmed to anticipate any fear and pain of child birthing as in our modern societies. Home birthing is becoming very popular in the world, if there are no known risk factors involved in the pregnancy and anticipated in the delivery. While the infant mortality rate of newborns in the USA is high, the infant mortality rate with midwives is extremely low.

The birthing process is a major stressor for most newborns. Many problems result from the lack of oxygen at birth caused by the cord being wrapped around the neck. Another possible problem is that the cord can be cut too soon before the baby has started to breath on its own. The baby can receive oxygen through the cord for 30 minutes, so the breathing passage needs to be cleared first.

If we eliminate fear and help the mother to give birth in a natural way, we can eliminate so much unnecessary stress and damage that are programmed into a child at birth.

INNER KNOWING AND EQUALITY

Within each one of us, we have a very special gift. It is that small, still voice. When we listen to it, it is never wrong. Some refer to it as intuition. It's that knowing what to do when we don't know what to do. We can always ask the advice of others, but we somehow have the correct answer to questions within ourselves.

We need to follow this inner knowing. When we defer to people outside ourselves for our answers, we can lose touch with our inner knowing. It may be beneficial to get many viewpoints on a given question, but the best answer is usually inside. We can get in touch with our inner knowing by stilling our minds and stopping the inner chatter that drowns out the small, still voice. How many times do we take the advice of others and not follow our inner guidance, only to realize that we would have been right had we followed our intuition? Even before the facility of language, we had an inner knowing. Tiny children can be role models in that they are so perceptive and aware, as we will discuss later.

How do we define equality? Of course we are all different, but we are all equal in that we are all human beings and deserve the respect and honor of existing as a human being. We may all be different with different abilities, genetics, interests, structures, races, skin colors, cultures, but we are all humans in the family of humanity.

CHILD/TEACHER/PARENT RELATIONSHIPS

Our children born today are quite evolved. Doesn't it seem like they are much smarter than we were at their age? When I look at my little granddaughter and compare her with my own children who were very bright, she is clearly even more evolved. Today's children are truly special and it is our responsibility to prepare a loving, challenging, clear environment for them. They know who they are and what they want. We must recognize them and celebrate their unique qualities and give them special loving care.

One hundred years ago, Dr. Maria Montessori, a physician turned outstanding pedagogue, recognized the innate abilities of children that would develop if they were only given an opportunity to learn. She taught that 80 per cent of all learning occurs before age six years. Now the researchers are saying that happens before age three! This period is when the brain connections are made. The child learns to walk, talk and forms major beliefs about himself/herself and the world. Thus, the parent has an enormous responsibility even before the child goes to preschool. They are like little sponges taking in everything they observe and experience. They are looking to adults as role models. They imitate our behavior.

We have been taught to live in fear, which is not to be confused with the respect for physical laws such as gravity. How would it look if we lived in acceptance? Most people have a great fear of loss.

At age four, children may be forced into competitive sports by some parents. We live in a competitive world where we learn that the most clever, most fit, most powerful and strongest will survive. So, we may strive to achieve the highest goals. However, we fall short, because everyone, in those terms, cannot be the most clever, most fit, strongest, nor most powerful. We are discouraged when we do not measure up to those standards in competition. Therefore we do not love ourselves as a result, because we are not number one! How can we all be number one? Did you ever really talk with someone who has lost the race, didn't win the gold medal, and didn't "win" the top score in the class? That, good people, is the majority of the world!

After decades of working with thousands of clients and students, I find that when an individual does not love, honor and respect themselves, the physical, mental, emotional, and spiritual selves suffer greatly.

Individuals are so busy trying to please others and compete with others, that they lose track of who they are and what they want for themselves in life.

The basis of competition can be to get more energy from another source. Energy comes in many forms: sunlight, oil, water, food, minerals, precious gems, money, and so on. If we are out of balance, we feel that we can never have enough energy, so we have to take it from others. This may be done openly, as in war, or quietly, as in the recent financial scandals. It may be done on a large scale or on a small scale. It may be done individually or collectively. This manifests in greed, which is an obsession. The secret we have missed is this: there is enough energy on the planet for all of us to live in relative abundance.

What affects one human being affects us all on some level and to some degree. A chain is only as strong as its weakest link. Competition leaves losers in a derelict status without basic needs having been met. Ramifications of the poverty status lead to misery, crime, and in general, an unnatural state of being. This affects all of humanity, each of us, in the long run.

What we can realize is that we are all different, with different talents, abilities, interests and life missions. No one can be the best you that you can be! No one can be the best person that your friend can be. You are not "that" individual. You are you! Together we make up a colorful, spectacular mosaic of the family of humanity. When we choose love and acceptance over fear, for ourselves and toward others, everyone wins and everyone succeeds. Just be the greatest you that you can be!

Every action taken by humans is either love-based (acceptance) or fear-based. People are always checking out what the competition is doing. Think of all the time, money and energy that are wasted on this joyless exercise of competition. Politics is a prime example. Has it really worked in the past? Has it brought us to a loving situation on the planet? Have we learned to live harmoniously in a family of humanity? Is the world free from fear? What society in the world is a model of coopera-tion, peace and acceptance? What country is free from crime, poverty, and ignorance?

Our governments keep making more laws and collecting more money, but our societies keep deteriorating. Should competition be with ourselves to be the best person we can be for ourselves? How does fear of success or failure, according to someone else's standards and control put limitations on you today?

When a child is born, s/he is basically free of most fears depending on the prenatal/natal process. S/he quickly imprints that the world is safe even with moments of danger, or that the world is dangerous.

When a two-year-old girl with her father visited our Montessori preschool with only the adult teachers present, she was so secure that she told her father to leave. She did not need him there in spite of the totally new environment and teachers. That same child on the first day of school, chose to ride the big bus with the other children, other parents and teacher, without her parents (and this in a new, foreign country). This child had had a home birth, natural care, bonded with her parents and had never been instilled with irrational fears. She could feel that this environment and the world were safe. She had a sense of what was safe, demonstrated in her happy acceptance of new things, new people.

Although a newborn is dependent on his/her environment, physical respect for physical laws is necessary to learn, but psychological fear can be crippling. For example, a baby is not born with the fear of public speaking. They are not concerned with who is listening or what that person's reaction may be -- until they are programmed otherwise. If they are punished for expressing, they will develop a fear of expression. Revisit your fears of early childhood. Are they still controlling you today?

Loving parents teach their children love and acceptance naturally. The basic family unit is a secure place for nurturing and protecting when they are young. When death or divorce is the situation, it is important to still have that loving environment for the children. When you know that your parents or caregivers love you, you will not feel the deep separation which children in orphanages or from dysfunctional homes feel. For parents to be indifferent to a child's needs is giving him/her the message that s/he is not essential and important.

When fear overtakes us, it cuts off the flow of love and acceptance. It numbs us, even physically in our bodies. Without acceptance of ourselves and acceptance of others, life is a difficult experience. Everywhere we turn, we face our limitations because of our fears. Then we wonder why we have to struggle so much in life rather than spreading happy wings to fly!

Parenting-issue fears can be a problem because of a child's association with substitute parents such as older siblings as well as caregivers. How has the placement in your family affected these issues? Did an older sibling terrorize you -- or comfort you?

What fears have you acquired as a result of your interactions with your parents, siblings and caregivers going back to a very early age? Again, get in touch with the situations, emotions, and feelings in your body. What did you learn from that situation? How has it limited you in life? How will your life be different if you no longer harbor that fear?

How much of our education is fear-based? What did you learn out of fear: fear of a teacher, fear of failing an exam, fear of looking stupid, fear of performing in public? How much do our children learn today because of the joy and desire to learn? When in the midst of taking final exams, I can tell you that very few of them study out of the love to learn that material.

In most Eastern European nations, all the students had to learn Russian under the Communist regime. A large number of these people can now hardly remember one word in Russian. Because they were blocked on the fear associated with the Russian language, they cannot benefit from the all those years of study of the language.

With fear in the way, we cannot live in the present time and enjoy the here and now. We pull in all the past negative experiences on the issue before us which negates our ability to absorb it, to learn from it.

Are there curriculums in today's schools which teach children awareness, honesty and responsibility? What good are some of the facts that we teach our children if they have no use for them in practical life? Can we teach children how to solve problems without violence, how to live without fear, how to love unconditionally, without prejudice? What adults have the following attributes? Where can we learn them? They are all within us to be uncovered, like a jewel that must be polished to bring out its brilliance. The following list are some of the essential values we must teach our children so that they may create a world of peace and love:

1. Critical Thinking
2. Inner Power versus Outer Force Understanding
3. Solving Problems Peacefully
4. Developing Relationships of Acceptance, Love
5. Self-development
6. Creative Expression
7. Awareness
8. Honesty and Fairness
9. Patience and Tolerance
10. Responsibility
11. Respecting Self and Others
12. Connection, Functions: Body, Mind and Spirit

The Montessori Method teaches concepts for living at a very early, tender age, when children are the most impressionable. It has children explore values, learn how to use them, apply them, question and live them! In Montessori the emphasis is on developing wisdom, not memorizing data (simply to regurgitate it) and that is why the children are so happy there.

Children resonate to the truth. This method of learning is in harmony with their very nature. Shall we give our children only knowledge or shall we give them wisdom, the tools to live an abundant, happy, productive, creative life? Search for, learn and use what works best!

PERSONAL RELATIONSHIPS

How many personal relationships are based on fear rather than love and acceptance? It may be fear of losing that person through separation, divorce or death, fear of loss of physical, emotional or economic support. When we doubt and distrust someone we love, it is a mirror of our own fear. The trauma and survival threats of childhood may still be with us. Our parents set the scene for our attitudes toward primary relationships and authority figures.

How have you internalized your parent's relationship? How are you following their pattern? What fears, addictions or obsessions did you develop as a result of their model (or lack of it)? Were these models based on betrayal, or perhaps abuse: physical, emotional, sexual, mental? Did your parents display a loving touch and loving glance often? What conditions did they have on that relationship? Did they stay committed? What underlying expectations and conditions do we have with the words, "I love you"? Silently do we express these conditions as "If you do as I want…If you change…If you do not change…If you rescue me…?

What were the underlying reasons that you chose that relationship? In the past, many women chose a husband for financial and physical security and many men chose a wife for convenient sex. That is all changing today as women are becoming more independent financially. Partners are marrying later and choosing a partner for compatibility, for sharing similar life goals, attitudes and interests. They can thus support each other in their lives, emotionally, spiritually, as well as in other ways.

~

One way to improve a relationship: A male student in Prague was soon to celebrate his 25th wedding anniversary, but had a problem. Eight years earlier his wife had banned him from sleeping with her because of his snoring. His roommate at the seminar commented that he sounded like a freight train. He volunteered for a correction on stage for snoring during one of my seminars. The next day, his roommate announced it had been a very quiet night. Hopefully, he enjoyed his 25th anniversary and his wife could now invite him back into the bedroom.

COMMUNITY RELATIONSHIPS

Which nation will rise up without fear and be a shining model for the world? This must all happen first within each individual heart. As individuals, we must get rid of our fear and pain as we clear the path for creating a society, which is also free of fear and pain. To replace fear, we have the acceptance/love model for our blueprint. The problem we have is with the Golden Rule: "Do unto others as you would have them do unto you." Why? Is it for the reason that we don't love and accept ourselves? So why can't we love and accept all manner of men/women and treat ourselves and the others with dignity and respect?

It is said that you can tell the level of a society by the way they treat the very young and the very old. Do we have a model society in the world from which we can learn? How do we internalize the responsibilities in a society? How effective and appropriate are the common laws of that society? Do the laws need changing or simplifying? Do we fear policemen and tax authorities or respect them? Are politicians our servants representing our collective best interests or are they our enemies? Do they respect you? Are students and teachers, employers and employees, respecting each other and treating each other with dignity? Why not? Can we work together to create a win-win situation for all? The way to acceptance and peace on earth begins as an inside job: inside each one of us. That is what my work is about!

Our societies re-program us to feel we must have certain things in life: a big home, luxury cars, many university degrees, and so on. So we must "do" certain work to obtain these things -- like working in a 9-5 job we hate. Then, when we "have" these things, we can "be" someone.

The reverse is that we can just "be" who we are, therefore "do" what we are happy working at and then we will naturally "have" what we need. At that point, we will be "on our place" in the world.

CHAPTER 5

SEXUAL CHALLENGES

MANY couples have come to me who have wanted to have a child and had no luck. They have tried various hormone therapies without success. The first order is to check for any emotional blockages. In one instance, when we went back to age five, my client recalled that she had a baby brother appear in the household suddenly, a stranger to her! Her parents had not prepared her at all for the event.

The programming was there on a very deep level. During our private session, she said to me, "I don't want a stranger in my body"! Apparently this surfaced from the subconscious level. We worked with getting the stress off the situation from when she was five. Subsequently, the emotional basis creating stress that caused the hormonal disturbances was cleared. Of course, me being a teacher, I pointed out that they must do their homework!

~

Last year I received the following email, "Dear Carol, I met with you in December 2006 because I and my husband wanted a baby, and we had several serious problems before meeting with you. I am happy to inform you that our son Andrew Greg was born 9th August in 2007. I would like to say many, many thanks for your help." I have received this same type of report from many couples with whom I have worked. One student was ten years without a child and within two years of our unblocking, she had her first child.

~

Many partners or couples schedule a meeting with me who are having difficulty in enjoying their sexual life. One student with whom I worked had no sexual pleasure in five years of marriage. We had to go to nine years of age where she and her brother were playing and he brushed her breast. She felt deep guilt which we released during our session. The next morning her husband sent me a huge bouquet of flowers!

~

One student wanted to work on her lack of sexual satisfaction. We went back to the birth process when the doctor told her mother to stop the labor because they were not ready. She stopped it somehow. Three hours later the doctor was shouting for her to start the labor again or they would lose the baby, but she could not. Then the doctor instructed a large assistant to get on top of her and bounce up and down on her abdomen. When the baby was born, she was black and blue with bruises. The position and movement during sex is somewhat similar, hence the trauma association and rejection of the act as an adult. What relief our student felt after that session.

~

Some of the deep emotional causes of sexual problems may be incest and rape. A very large number of women (and men) have been sexually molested at an early age or abused later sexually, frequently by a family member or trusted friend. Children are very reluctant to tell their parents because they are made to feel as though they have created the situation and therefore feel deep guilt. I have found that these situations have caused deep scars that can be released, sometimes in one session. But, forgiveness is key, mostly forgiving themselves and also the other person involved. Re-establishing self-esteem and therefore feelings of worth in being a female or male is paramount to the healing.

~

One client was very boyish, in her dress, style and mannerisms. She knew that her sister had been molested by their father for years, but she always managed to escape. Was her boyish cover-up a kind of perceived protection?

~

A client had a swollen prostate and was on medication, but still got up several times during the night to urinate. We returned to age of cause at 23 when he felt his wife did not enjoy their sex life. His prostate is now functioning normally.

~

A student in Moscow volunteered to work on her relationship with her husband during a seminar. She lived in Moscow with their daughter and her husband lived in St. Petersburg with their son. She knew from her early history that at her conception her mother was in a detention camp and while interred there had been raped by a soldier (her father). We were all surprised at the anger that surfaced in her during the session as she said she would like to get a pair of scissors and cut him to pieces! She was furious! Her anger had transferred itself to all men in general. After the session, she had a lot of positive energy unblocked, so we told the gentlemen in the class to be careful!

~

A 20-year old man came to a private session because of a problem with his prostate and with stuttering. His mother did everything for him, including answering his questions during the session. He had never touched a girl, not even to hold her hand. He does not go out unless he is with his mother.

When a therapist suggested that he take supplements for the prostate, his mother said that she had choked on a pill one time, so she no longer takes any pills. Of course she would never allow her son to take pills for fear that he may choke.

The big issue was the addiction to the mother -- or vice versa. One is there to give out the pain, and the other is there to receive it! By age 20, the pattern of addiction to the mother may be so very deeply ingrained. This can profoundly affect a child's psyche in areas of their later sexual life, their self esteem, their interpersonal relationships, making choices, being responsible and independent.

Dependency started at a very early age and has been layered over by many events that damaged this young person profoundly. The fears of the mother can be transferred to the fetus even starting in the womb. If he is to get better, the mother needs very serious work especially if this young person continues living with her. It may take many sessions for both of them. How much influence does a mother have on the son's male self image? Can she emasculate him?

At age four this same young man was bitten by a dog. He then began stuttering. I have found many speech problems in cases where children were attacked by a dog, a truly frightening event. Most of these problems are settled in one session. This young man has many deep issues to view and resolve.

~

For three years a young lady and her husband wanted to have a baby. Her doctor told her that her level of prolactin was too high. He put her on hormone treatment. She has been emotionally upset since she has been on this medication. Now her doctor told her the problem was stress related and that she should see a psychologist. At this time she came to see me, having heard of the success I have had with other cases of women wanting to become pregnant.

At age three her brother was conceived and she was very excited and wanted him. However, when he arrived home, all the family was gathered around his crib and she was behind them. Her parents told her the story of a time when her father was holding her brother. She looked at her father with very demanding eyes and said, "Put down the baby!" The parents tried to explain to her that they had to take care of the baby as they did when she was a baby, but she was hurt and didn't want to hear that. From a very early age and for the next 12 years she felt excluded and ostracized from the family. She was no longer the center stage person.

During the session, she realized how deeply her brother's birth had affected her whole life. She was now ready to let go of that stress and move forward, welcoming a new little soul, her own child, into her family.

~

Many young ladies who have had problems with menses: lack of, painful, or irregular periods, have benefited from my work. Such problems as Candida have corrected when we dealt with the emotional cause. As I have stated earlier, stress causes a shutdown in the energy flow to specific organs and systems so that the energy does not get carried to a specific part of the body and toxins do not get released. We are usually able to change this energy flow.

CHAPTER 6

LEARNING CHALLENGES

W HAT is dyslexia and how can it be corrected? In the past, as well as in the present and by many professionals, dyslexia has been defined as an incurable disease with the prognosis being dim. People are told they must learn to live with it, to cope and to tell those they meet that they are dyslexic.

The concept with which we work is a very different approach. We believe that dyslexia is not a disease, that most of the learning blocks, which are called dyslexia, can be removed. Our results also prove this with a very high success rate, usually a complete reversal of the dyslexic condition.

We work with the concept that when stress overloads the organism, it goes into the overwhelm mode and programs in a neurological blind spot in order to survive. This interrupts the normal neurological flow. When the same or a similar situation presents itself again, the conscious thinking area of the brain will take the incoming data, compare it with what has happened in the past and then the person will have a specific reaction, usually repeating the past reaction, which becomes a pattern in a future similar situation.

An example of this reaction could be that ten-year old David gets up to read aloud in front of the class. Reading has to be one of the most difficult processes of the young child. Numerous coordinating activities must be synchronized in the brain and body to make reading possible.

Let us imagine that David comes upon some new words, which he does not recognize and he does not know how to pronounce. If he were at home he could ask his parents for help. At his desk in school, he could ask a friend or the teacher. However, he is called upon to read in front of the class. He must read perfectly now.

Since he does not know some new words, he guesses and they are wrong. The other children laugh because it sounds funny and perhaps the teacher makes a comment. The very delicate eye muscles may be affected by the stress hormones which are now, instantly emitted. David sits down, embarrassed and flushed. He realizes that he has failed, failed to meet others' expectations and failed to meet his own.

The next time he is called upon to read, his body/brain remembers that experience, either consciously or subconsciously, and that embarrassed, flushed feeling goes throughout his body even before he stands up to read. He is so nervous. The stress hormones go on again affecting the delicate eye muscles (or any other area such as the voice). He cannot differentiate among the printed symbols, so he guesses and again it is incorrect. Maybe the children don't laugh this time and maybe the teacher doesn't make a comment, but he knows. He has failed again.

So the label "dyslexic" is assigned, a label that he will wear the rest of his life and one that will continue to affect everything he does. When he is 45 years old, he may not remember the original cause of his problem. But the memory is stored in his brain/body that will cause the same reaction each time he attempts to read, as when he was ten years old.

When we were very young children, we were required to meet our parents' expectations of perfection and performance, according to their standards. Later, many adults and our peers had certain expectations of us. Perhaps some of these expectations were beyond our capabilities, interests and needs. However, we knew we had to meet these standards whether we wanted to or not. We were required to study subjects we were not interested in and that had no relevance or application to our life then or since. We had to do endless, mindless drill work and had our creativity and individuality stifled. We had to be a different person for different peoples' expectations and we lost our own true personality in the process of trying to please everyone around us.

By denying our own needs and interests, we became those expectations. Thus, these experiences in life were stress-producing, which led to the creation of many of our dyslexic blind spots.

Under stress we have diminished awareness which can be labeled dyslexia. Stress not only affects our ability to learn, but it permeates areas of our lives such as relationships, health, finances, careers, self-esteem, including many areas of our mental, physical, emotional, and spiritual well being.

Our daily lives are filled with challenges. How do we handle them? The amount of negative stress we generate on a given challenge tells us how we have handled that challenge. When we go into confusion, worry and despair on an issue, we are functioning out of fear, pain and fear of pain and do not see positive solutions for that problem. So, in reality: it's not the problem that's the problem, but how we feel about the problem that's the problem.

If there is an extended delay at the airport, someone could have a heart attack because of the worry of missing a very important meeting on the other end. Another person would call ahead and advise his colleagues what to do and then buy a great book he has wanted to read, find a quiet, comfortable spot and have a nice extended vacation.

When we get the stress off the situation of the past, which is controlling us today because of the fear, pain and fear of pain from the past, then we are "at choice" in the moment. We are then free to choose a new appropriate action, rather than a painful repetition of the past: a reaction.

Through stress testing, which is similar to biofeedback, we are able to access the stress-causing incident that took only three seconds to program in as a blind spot. Then, with very gentle exercises, we are able to reconnect the neurological flow and the body/brain returns to its normal balance. So stress diminishes our awareness, thus causing learning blocks.

The body is a great tool for giving us information (via a reaction) at the time of an experience. The body records everything we think, do and say, as well as what happened to us and how we felt about it all.

An obvious example of this messaging is blushing. If a painful, embarrassing moment is recalled on any level, the person has no control over this bodily reaction.

~

One August a ten-year old was brought to me for a session. She was told that she must go into the class for slow learners. She had not done well that year in school and scored one and a half years below grade level on her standardized tests. The cause of the problem happened on her tenth birthday when her mother gave her a favorite ring from when she, the mother, was also ten. Her daughter lost the ring that same day!

When I tested her, she could not focus when looking down. On the day she had been looking down for the ring on the ground, she felt fear, disappointment: stress. This persisted whenever she looked down thereafter (as in taking a test or doing homework). After the correction she returned to school and retook the test and scored one and a half years <u>above</u> grade level (an improvement total of three grades!), was left in the normal class and lived happily ever after. But think of what could have happened to this young lady's future if she had not been corrected and had moved to the slower class!

~

A young engineer wanted to move to Berlin from Budapest. The new job required that he know German. Since it was his mother's dream that he learn German, she provided German lessons starting at age six and throughout his education. It did not stick! So, back to age five we went with him. At that time there was very little Hungarian television, but they could receive many Austrian programs in German. This little guy was so frustrated that he could not understand these programs that he decided he did not like that foreign language! After his session, all that is now changed. He has three more months to master German. I am confident that he will pass that exam.

~

In the school for slow learners in Budapest, my graduates and I worked with 80 children. Little first grader Kati would not participate in school and not much else in life. Her father reported that she was sad and withdrawn. I found that her mother had passed away when she was four. At that time she constructed an internal wall to protect herself from more pain. After three sessions, she became open, vibrant, did well in school and in social encounters. After a lecture there for the teachers and parents, her father came to me with tears in his eyes and said, "Thank you for giving me my little girl back". Kati is now a young adult and the last I heard, a few years ago, was progressing nicely. Her results are included in the following report with a summary of the work with those children as compiled by the school principal:

BUDAPEST RESEARCH REPORT NOVEMBER, 1996-MARCH: 1997

In November 1996, a project to help children and do research was initiated by Carol Ann Hontz and several of her graduate facilitators in a school for children with special problems. The location of the school is in a housing project with many elderly citizens, with high unemployment and with social and financial problems in this district. This influences the operation of the school and its profile. The factors of the environment were one of the reasons why this location was chosen.

At this school there are two special classes for learning-disabled children with a limited number of children per class. The teachers are trained to work with disabled children. Three categories of children were identified for the project:

1. Learning-disabled: dyslexic, dysgraphic, dyscalculate, poor concentration and poor coordination.

2. Problematic: difficulties in social interaction and communication with teachers and other students, defiance, inattentiveness in their classes.

3. Psychological: focus on failure, phobias, introversion, very loud, aggressive behavior. Some are victims of child abuse.

Each child was recommended by the teacher or it was requested by the parents to have stress-release sessions. The plan was to have three individual sessions and then re-evaluate. The sessions were done with children from the first, second, fourth and seventh classes. Eighty children were involved in the project.

A psychological appraisal was written about the students in these special classes which was compared with the teachers' and parents' opinion. This team of parents, teachers and the psychologist reported the following information:

"After the first stress-release sessions, we could see remarkable changes in 80% of the cases. In 10%, we did not see outer changes and with the last 10%, the children did not have the last three sessions. If the child goes back to the home environment of child abuse, alcoholic parents, etc., then more problems are being constantly created".

The leaders of the school held a parents' meeting when parents were informed about the results. The parents were very happy to speak about their children's progress and were so pleased that there was help for their children. More and more parents are asking for stress-release sessions for their other children, as well as the school children, as they see the amazing results of their classmates. Below are several case studies from the eighty students as reported by their teachers and verified by head-mistress of the school, Dr. Marika Kelemen:

"K.D. first class (six year old), dyslexic class:
    After the first stress-release session, no change could be noticed. After the second and third sessions, major differences could be seen in her behavior. She had been sad, distressed, depressed. Her mother died when she was four years old. This child never wanted to participate in the

lessons and was very silent at home. The speech therapist's report: "Slow psychological rhythm, low level of ability and production". After the three sessions she became totally free and happy. She seemed to be flying through the air, she is so enthusiastic about her lessons and her personality has completely changed. Her father said she has been reborn! Her results are better and better.

A.T. first class (six year old), dyslexic class:

After birth, several deficiencies emerged. The speech therapist's opinion: "He has problems with vision, word and text comprehension, memory, concentration, is two years retarded as compared with his age group". His parents said that changes could already be detected after the first session. He is now more active, able to count much better, recognizes figures and comprehension of texts is good. He is enthusiastic and active during lessons.

M. Sz. (six year old), dyslexic class:

He was described as not a peaceful child who does not pay attention. He is angry with the world. He can say long words only by slowly sounding them out in syllables. Teacher's report: "After his sessions, he is more calm and patient and communication is possible with him".

T.M. (six year old), dyslexic class:

He has problems with adapting socially. He does not participate in class, his behavior is passive and he smiles on such occasions. The huge progress experienced after the session was followed by a return to his former state, perhaps due to his home environment or the need for more sessions.

G.S. (six year old), dyslexic class:

Speech therapist's evaluation: "His speech is difficult to

understand, his articulation is bad. It is difficult for him to express his thoughts. His movements are not coordinated. After the stress-release session: "He is more resolved and calm, his walk is more balanced".

A.T. (six year old) dyslexic class:

According to the opinion of the teachers, he was difficult to get along with, was not interested and was easily offended. He had tremendous fear and got tense when the teacher appeared. He was rude to the others and behaved harshly. After the second session, he is already polite and neat, nice and more calm, and very active during the lessons. After the third session, he is in the sky, rarely gets offended, but calms down fast in such cases. Three months after the first session, he still expresses fear toward one of his relatives.

H.E. (seven year old):

He had been seriously afraid of water. The gymnastics lessons are held in a swimming pool. (This problem emerged in the case of several students.) After two or three sessions, he has looked forward to the swimming lesson, and after the fourth session he swam without any auxiliary equipment. He is pleased to swim now and does not have to be "ill" at that time.

E.K. (eight years old):

He tries to avoid all failures by getting "sick". He was afraid of swimming as well. After the fourth session, he went into deep water and is making nice progress in swimming. He does not get sick now and the progress in learning can also be seen.

A.F. (seven year old):

His speech is affected and his movements are uncoordinated.

Since the stress-release sessions, his movement has visibly improved and he has made significant progress in swimming. His speaking abilities have shown some improvement.

P.M. (ten year old):
He has forgotten his homework and has poor comprehension. After three stress-release sessions, his text comprehension has improved and he now prepares his homework.

D.K. (ten year old):
Although he is a boy, he behaved as a girl. He spoke in a posed way and was bashful. After the sessions, spectacular improvement has been experienced. He no longer speaks in the posed way and his behavior has become more normal.

V.Gy. (ten year old):
His performance in math was very low. After the sessions, he started to work slowly, but surely, alone and at an acceptable level.

IN CONCLUSION

Most of the other students not described above who have been stress-released have become more balanced, calm and are participating more at their lessons. They are involved more in their work. Their attention span is better.

Most children, even after one session, had the following behavioral changes: improvement in reading, counting and speaking skills, more balanced movements, ceasing of bad headaches, and disappearance of phobias such as fear of water.

Because of the high success rate of the program at this school, the teachers' interest was keen in this process, so two brief courses were organized and taught to them by Carol Ann Hontz. The goal of these courses was twofold: (1) To give the teachers the beginning basic skills to help their students and just as importantly, (2) to have the teachers acquire a deep understanding of the mental, physical and emotional development of the child as it relates to his environment from the home and at school. Learning disabilities, as well as most problems, are created by stress when the organism cannot deal with any more pain and fear and the system goes into overwhelm causing blockages in favor of survival. The individual creates a blind spot with an interruption in the natural neurological flow. This can easily be corrected by simple, gentle, non-invasive exercises and techniques.

Many of the teachers in this school are now regularly doing certain fun exercises with their classes, such as the cross crawl and the infinity tracing. They report that just minutes of practice has a great influence on the effectiveness of their lesson. These exercises are illustrated and explained in "Inner Treasures", a book written for children of all ages by Carol Ann Hontz.

Children are our most precious natural resource. The home, the school, the community, the governments and all of society must work together to provide a high quality of education and a positive home environment to prepare our children for a higher quality of life where they can become more self-sufficient, peaceful, creative, happy, purposeful, and fulfilled in life."

April 26, 1997
Dr. Marika Kelemen

The day after his session for reading/writing, I received this message from this first grade child's mother:

"Usually, his teacher would write about frustrations my son was experiencing when reading and how we should continue to work with him." The day after the session the teacher wrote: "Your son was more on track today and read a page from the story we were reading, pretty well. He had trouble with only one or two words and was more fluent. He paid attention, tracking the words as we read the entire story."

Months later, I talked with him and he is enjoying reading this summer. Also, his mother said that he has become so very social and loved by everyone, a new experience in his life!

~

Following is a mother's story of a young client who is now a teenager:

"My son was born in 1991 with a long labor because of a breech position, ending with a c-section. Because of what the doctors said was a deprivation of oxygen, he had severe brain damage. The prognosis from a top specialist doctor told me that he would never walk. His back and abdominal muscles were very weak. I was told by this specialist that he would always be in a wheelchair. Because he couldn't stand and climb alone, I took him for manual therapy and at ten months, he stood alone. At one and a half years he walked and spoke some words. At age two, he started to put together sentences. At age four and a half he entered Carol's Montessori Preschool and Carol did private sessions with him. This environment was the best atmosphere for him where he gained self-confidence and could develop a healthy mental attitude. Around this age his IQ was tested at 54. He underwent re-patterning (a movement to balance right and left hemispheres of the body as taught by Carol) for two years, once per week. Now, his speech is normal, his IQ is 72, his co-ordination is nearly normal; he skis and swims. Through these various stress releases and exercises, his improvement has been very good and we continue to help him in various ways. I am a medical doctor."

Note: I saw this child a couple of times per year and he continued to improve.

~

Another student is a famous actress and had a major reading block. She would have to go into the forest with complete silence to memorize her lines for seven hours a day. Great trepidation clouded her life over this situation. After the class demonstration she could read perfectly. So many of these blocks go back to a situation in school and can be released easily.

~

A client related that she had never been able to hear with her left ear. We went back to age six weeks in the womb where her mother "did not want to hear" that she was pregnant.

This was her note afterward:

"I still am in somewhat of a state of disbelief and shock with how you were able to get my left ear to hear for the first time in my whole life! My ear keeps hearing more clearly. I cried after yoga class (tears of joy) because I could really HEAR THE BIRDS singing during the meditation! I remember you telling me another person you cleared was happy to hear them. I guess I never thought about it until I heard the birds TWICE as loud as ever in 50 years! What can I possibly say to thank you enough?" She also said she can now choose which ear to use with the telephone.

Earlier she had written:

"On a personal level in my private sessions with Carol, we uncovered some tragic moments in my life which continually kept me beating myself up and feeling unworthy. Carol gently led me to feel forgiveness and compassion for myself and others, back to a state of grace. Of course, being human, there will always be dragons to slay. When I was first introduced to Carol I had had an accident and was in a very dark place. After she worked with me, I felt the anguish release. Now that dark memory has no hold on me. I cannot wait to continue working with her techniques to help unleash my unlimited potential!"

~

One student in our seminar had a 58 per cent hearing loss, and her husband had nearly the same. She related that now she understood why her daughter commented that she didn't know why mom and dad always shouted at each other!

We were able to correct the stress of what the mother did not want to hear at a certain age and her hearing was restored during the session in class. That evening she went home and corrected her husband with the correction she had learned that day in our seminar! Their home is much quieter now.

~

During a television show in Budapest, I stress released a gentleman who volunteered for a demonstration. He had both vision and hearing problems after being hit by a car. We did the research: just minutes before the accident he had a fight with his wife. He was blind with rage and did not want to hear what she had to say. He went storming out of their apartment and did not see or hear the car which hit him.

It was not the accident, but the earlier argument that caused the hearing loss and vision problem! After our session, he had a very measurable change in his vision and hearing. You may have heard the expression, "blind with rage" and "to turn a deaf ear". What do you not want to see or hear?

~

Earlier in one of our first courses in Budapest, a student volunteered for the balancing of the hemispheres correction. The left brain is in charge of our logic, detail, math, judgment, fear, time, and it is the control center for the right side of our bodies. The right side is our dreamer side, infinite possibilities, art, sees the whole picture, timeless, fearless, non-judgmental, and it controls the left side of the body. When both hemispheres are working, we have good coordination and function well in all those areas. If we are stressed, we can shut down some areas of the brain at certain times and the result may be a problem with one of those hemispheric functions which can affect coordination.

This student's coordination was extremely poor. She could not learn to swim or ride a bike. Her walking was quite awkward and unbalanced. She could not drive because she would switch on her left-turn signal and then proceed to turn right, a rather dangerous mix-up! We researched the cause to when her mother threw her into the Danube River when she was a few months old and her father rescued her! I can still see her that day in the classroom walking suddenly with the greatest of ease, grace and poise. What a total transformation, a very real metamorphosis in her life at age 42!

~

In a lecture in Budapest a 65-year old woman volunteered for the reading correction demonstration. She had never been able to read well. She reads well now! What a joy it is to help people change their lives so dramatically and so very gently!

CHAPTER 7

ALLERGIES

WHEN our body is chemically imbalanced, we may need more or less of a substance in our body. However, there are times when major stress has occurred at the time we were eating a certain food, smelling a specific odor, experiencing some sensation. We may then program in an allergic reaction when we experience that sensation again. This is true of many food allergies.

The base-line with these "emotional" allergies is rejection of self or others. A good example is an allergy to flowers. Funerals are a very emotional time for most people and there are usually lots of flowers there. Consequently, flowers can be associated with the pain of loss or perhaps fear of death. Many food allergies stem from children being forced to eat certain foods. People can have an allergic reaction to so many things: plants, animals, people, perfumes, locations, the sun, wind, rain, snow, fabrics, plastics, medications, food. Some individuals are "universal reactors", that is, people who are allergic to many things.

MILK ALLERGY

A message from one of my students:

"My sister was allergic to milk. She was taken to the hospital several times and had many difficulties because of this illness. She could not eat anything which contained milk. She had only one single session with Carol and that evening she could drink milk without having any problem. All the problems she had with milk in the last 15 years simply disappeared that day…and it is not magic, it is Carol's wonderful work."

This is her version of the story of her milk allergy:

"One day, when I was 17, my stomach started cramping with a strong pain. I had never felt this before. I had terrible pains. As it turned out, I couldn't eat anything which contains milk, milk sugar or butterfat (cream)--without having pains and cramps. I suffered from milk (lactose) allergy.

I lived with this problem for several years and many doctors analyzed me, however they couldn't help in any way. After a very thorough checkup in a hospital and trying out many special diets, the doctors finally told me that I should bow to it (accept it). I should live my whole life with having this illness, it won't expire.

A few weeks after having this final diagnosis, I met Carol. After talking with her about my problems I decided to try her treatments with kinesiology. I had only one session with Carol, where she found out (with her special muscle-testing method), that my allergy derived from a very bad experience in the elementary school when our teacher put me to shame in front of many children and parents. Carol made the correction and I went home. After having the treatment I felt very happy and energetic, and I felt I had lost a very heavy weight off my mind. My eyes glistened and I was really very happy. However I didn't think that anything had changed with my allergy. I made a test: I ate some sour cream in the evening and waited for the usual allergic reaction. However nothing happened! My allergy seemed to be over! Since then -- it was many years ago -- I have no more problems, so I don't need to deprive myself of any food or drink. Now I can eat and drink anything I want!

I'm very happy that I met Carol and I'm very thankful for her helping me. I have seen that the specialized kinesiology can really make our life much better. With my partner and some friends, we decided to attend some courses. These courses were held by Carol and we liked them very much! I think we learned very much from these courses and we can use this information in our life. Thanks to Carol for that!"

Later this lady had such a very strong allergic reaction to cosmetics that her face became extremely swollen so that she looked like a monster! We were able to correct the emotional cause and the swelling disappeared within 24 hours.

FISH ALLERGY

Another client was so allergic to fish. She could not tolerate the smell of fish or even the thought of fish. We found that age three was the root cause when her five-year old brother and his friend were chasing her around the house and beating her with a frozen fish! We released the stress and she gave a happy speech in our Toastmaster's Club about how that day had changed her life forever. It was not really the fish that was the problem -- but the rejection/teasing by her brother and friend.

FRAGRANCE ALLERGY

A student's comments:

"As I was driving home to Poulsbo Sunday after leaving all of you wonderful people, my glasses were bothering me. I would put them on and it would feel like they were someone else's! This is Tuesday evening and my glasses are too strong, so I have had a correction in vision. It is really driving me nuts because I am in between my glasses and 20/20. Luckily my eyes never were really bad because I can drive without them. But to read street signs, I have to be near them.

As you taught us to do, I tested what was affecting my eyes and it was an allergy to fragrances. When I get a whiff of a fragrance (except those that are still the way nature made them), I get a pain around my eyes. This has been going on as long as I can remember and I have worn glasses since age 15. I will keep you posted on progress. After my private sessions with you as well as your seminars, I was at a funeral with many people that I have known for years and everyone was telling me how great I looked. Thank you, Carol, for all of that!"

WEATHER ALLERGY

One recent student would get a sinus problem and headache if she sat in a draft or if a storm were coming. We had to research age five where she was playing in a mud puddle in the rain. Her mother scolded her and told her she would get sick if she went out in the storm. She was calm after the correction and we are optimistic about future storms in her life!

ALLERGY TO HOT PEPPERS

We went to lunch with a friend who was visiting from Prague. Since she was in Hungary, she wanted a typical Hungarian meal. However, she got more than she bargained for with that Hungarian meal! She cannot eat spicy food and was very careful to ask about ingredients. The waiter assured her that the dish she was ordering was not spicy. However, on the edge of her plate were a few fresh slices of the usual Hungarian hot pepper. Not knowing it was hot, she ate a bit. She could not put out the fire with bread or water; her lips began to swell; she was perspiring and feeling very distressed! She said, "I think I need an emergency session with you!"

We went back to age five when she was with her grandmother who was the only person she felt loved by, who cared for her and cooked for her. Her grandmother usually ate food prepared spicy hot. To please her grandma and get her approval, she ate the spicy food (that she really didn't like) and everything on her plate. Eating what other people wanted her to eat and eating everything on her plate became a pattern in her life.

We did the correction. Immediately the burning sensation was gone, the swelling receded and she was calm again. Later she put the peppers aside on another plate but rubbed her eye with the same fingers. Then we had the second spicy pepper problem! Her eyes began burning and tearing so profusely that she could not see! We again went back to age five, but this time later in that year when her beloved grandmother passed away. This, she did not want to "see" as she then felt alone in the world. This young lady rejected her own desires in order to please her grandmother. Again, the burning stopped (after the second correction).

ONION ALLERGY

One student was allergic to onions. Our research showed that when she was a teen, her father was striking her at the table when she was eating onions. After the session she was fine with onions.

ALLERGY TO PLANTS

An eight-year old client had allergies to plants, especially pollen. She also bit her nails. The father had left the mother when she knew she was pregnant. The father came back and then left again when the baby was eight months old. On the rare occasion that the father met with the mother and child, they (the parents) were often fighting. With the basis of rejection of self and others for allergies, we worked through this issue with her father and now she is allergy free.

~

Another individual was allergic to lots of stimuli in the outdoors. Each time he went outdoors, he had the symptoms of hay fever, especially in the summertime. Our research showed that at an early age his pet dog was killed on the road by a car and he watched it happen. After the session, his allergy was gone.

~

My business manager complained of her allergy acting up at the end of August. Her eyes were burning and itching. She thought it was related to pollen. We had to review age 13. What came immediately to mind was that she hated to be "penned in" at school and would make up any excuse to take a walk and have some peace away from sitting all day in a confined spot. She would find any excuse to get away for even 30 minutes. She always had the allergy in late August when school starts in Hungary! In her after-school, aftercare class, her teacher gave her permission to go to a shop to buy an exercise/writing book. The shop was closed, so she decided to go to a shop that was much further away. She walked slowly enjoying her freedom. Meanwhile her teacher became very worried and expressed that deep concern to my client upon her return which made her feel guilty.

My client said that she felt she was too independent, then and also now, and that "it hurts others". When I asked her how that relates to present time, she said that her son needed all his books to start school that morning. Since he did not use most of the exercise books from the previous year, she had saved things from last year. The only problem was that her younger son had "sold" them to his grandfather when he was "playing store" and grandpa was not yet awake next door to retrieve the books. Her son was upset that she had not taken care to get his books ready. Again, she felt guilty for not thinking of other people's needs, thereby hurting another person.

When she could forgive herself and learn to balance these situations, her allergy would be better. Allergy cause can be: rejection of self or others. Two days later I checked with her and the burning and itching in her eyes was still gone and should remain so since we have eliminated the emotional stress of the memory of the root cause.

~

My interpreter came to work and his nose was running like a faucet. He said that it happens the last two weeks of August so it must be due to some kind of pollen. We had to examine age three when he said he hated his brother so much that he wanted to push his eyes out. This hatred continued into adulthood and is only now abating. He always felt that his brother did not respect his privacy. At age three, he wanted to create a conspiracy with his mother against his brother and father. He had a water color set and told his mother that half of the colors represented him and his mother and the other half were his father and brother, as if the two color groups were enemies. I asked him how that relates to present time. He had issues with his brother and father all his life. He said he must keep his borders with his brother, but that it is time to stop being selfish and start taking others into consideration.

After he arrived at his home, he phoned to say that his nose stopped running, that he had a good night's sleep and the next day his nose was fine. He just had a bit of hoarseness. He also reported that he had had a fever during this time and felt that it was healing his body. Several days later he feels great. He is very happy that the two weeks of suffering every year are over.

ALLERGY TO PAINT

A 23-year old young man had three very serious coughing fits in the last few weeks. The intensity of the coughing was deep. His mother recommended that he come to me to work on his relationship with his father. He had gone to the doctor and had allergy tests that showed no trace of allergies. He had been painting cars with his father and the idea of an allergy to paint had come to his mind. He works with his father and they also restore cars as a hobby, working long hours and having little free time.

We had to go to age three when he remembered being told that he went to their cellar. He opened a can of paint and put his hand into it. He then put the paint into his eyes and had to be rushed to the hospital to have it flushed out. He also remembered a time at age ten when his father was painting. They had a problem because he said that his father was a hard man and they argued a lot.

My client now has little time for himself because his father is a workaholic and also expects him to be. His father helps him with his hobbies which includes race car driving, giving him tools, transportation and helps work on his cars. However, he must establish his borders with his father and communicate how he feels and what he wants, which he does not really do with most people.

When he asks his father for the night off to be with his friends, his father says nothing; he goes out and then feels guilty. We focused on his relationship with his father and on communication. That relationship should be different now as my client takes back his power and is expressing what he wants in his life. This correction will ripple out to his relationships with all his associates. He understands that he no longer needs to stifle those emotions but can express them. Then they will not show up later as dis-ease in his body! He can spread his wings and fly!

~

Countless students and clients, with our system, have been able to go back to the emotional cause -- rejection of self or others -- and be rid of allergies to food, animals, plants, weather, sun conditions, and so on, ending the years of suffering.

GLUTEN INTOLERANCE

With this client's gluten allergy, we researched age ten when his father was very strict and physically abusive. The young child always had the fear that his math and other work would not be good enough for his father. If one is eating something and has emotional stress at that specific time, he may become allergic to that food because of the association of the stress at the time of eating it. This was my client's email two weeks after his session:

"You may remember us. You helped us about two weeks ago. I myself have completely come out of the gluten intolerance and I just can't tell you what a great feeling it is. As for my wife, we don't know yet, but will keep you informed. I just want to say a real heartfelt thank you for your help with my allergy. It is such a wonderful thing to be eating normal food again and not suffering from all the stomach pain and other things." Note: I worked with this couple on stress with conceiving a child. It was as they were about to leave – as an afterthought -- that he mentioned his gluten intolerance. I spent only a few more minutes working with him -- with wonderfully satisfying results!

CHAPTER 8

COMPULSIVE BEHAVIOR

PSYCHOLOGICAL, SOCIAL, PHYSICAL PROBLEMS: ORIGINS OF ADDICTIONS

ADDICTIONS grow out of the fear of the past. They are an irrational dependence on a substance, object, person, place, an emotion such as perfectionism or anything that keeps us in present time feeling as good as we possibly can. We do not want to remember the fear and pain of the past. The cause may be on a deep subconscious level.

ALCOHOL ADDICTION

A big, 33-year old policeman from the Black Sea area came to me in Moscow to correct his addiction to alcohol, which was interfering with his job. We researched a time in kindergarten when he fell in love with a beautiful little girl. In the Russian school system at that time, children stayed overnight at kindergarten because the parents were working. These two children decided they would sleep together that night. As they were all cuddled up in each other's arms, the teacher saw them and punished them severely. Later their parents punished them.

As this policeman was telling me the story, the tears were streaming down his cheeks. He apologized because, he said, big boys don't cry.

I told him it was OK to let go of all that sadness. He said that he still remembered the little girl's name.

He never had a personal relationship after that, because he learned that if you really love someone you get punished for it. He replaced personal relationships with alcohol because the pain was so great from the past. If you're numb, supposedly you do not feel so much pain. We corrected the issue and before the seminar ended he had established a happy relationship with another student.

~

Many years ago a gentleman was about to have his first child, and he wanted to stop his addiction to alcohol. We had to go to the original cause at age three where he went to a beautiful preschool. He loved his preschool and the garden with the little fountain pool in the middle of the garden. However, this preschool closed and they moved his preschool down the street to a modern building. Every chance he got, he would escape and return to his former preschool and that beautiful garden.

When I saw the photo of him and his brother in the preschool he loved, I realized it was the same one which I then occupied with my Montessori Preschool! I told him he was welcome to visit us there any time he wished. The last time I heard, he was not over-indulging in alcohol anymore. What may seem so insignificant to us as adults can actually have created a lifetime problem, which began as a young child.

ADDICTION TO THINGS

Most things we do or don't do in life originate in compulsive behaviors. A friend insisted on keeping his tags on his suitcases from every trip he had taken. I discovered that the reason for this compulsive behavior was because, as a child, he was not allowed to go outside his family's property to play with other children and no other children were allowed in to play with him. In his long, adult lifetime he had lived in or traveled to more than 90 different countries, some many times! When we got in touch with the realization of why he compulsively had to prove that he could travel outside "his area", he immediately removed the tags from his bags.

~

One of my friends wanted to work on letting go of things, people, and old belief systems that were no longer benefiting her. We had to go to age three when she suddenly remembered that she lost her beautiful daisy pacifier. She was so very sad and would not accept a replacement. She pretended that it was OK, but she knew deep down in her heart it was not.

Bringing up that memory was still so sad and painful for her at age 28! She cried! Two years later she returned to that same situation, this time with letting go too quickly with her job and her primary relationships if they were too challenging. She needed to balance the "letting go" aspect. It was a matter of knowing when to let go, when to hold on, not too quickly or too slowly, but in a balanced way.

ADDICTION TO OVEREATING

Our reasons for compulsive behavior can run so deeply that, until we can connect with and release the cause, the compulsion controls us. Overeating can have many emotional roots. The following is one of fear of punishment:

At age ten, this boy had to finish everything on his plate. His mother was described by him as stern, aggressive and abusive. For example, he was served meat that was freezer-burned and which had a repulsive taste to him. Nevertheless, while crying and pleading not to have to eat the meat, he was made to sit at the dinner table until it was finished. Although his mother smiled and pretended to be happy with other people, to her son she often scowled and had a nasty look on her face.

Later in life he continued with the enforced obsession of not wasting food and would eat all on his plate even if he did not enjoy it. He felt that he was like his mother (stern, aggressive) but wanted to be gentle like his father whom he had seen only a few times in his lifetime.

We discussed his mother's difficult life being a single mom. We spoke of the abuse she must have received as a child which so often establishes the role model played out later in life. And, we discussed the positive things she did give him in life. Now he has more of an awareness of other people's reasons for doing what they do and is able to understand and forgive them and forgive himself as he forgave his mother. Goodbye to compulsive eating!

PROCRASTINATION

Countless clients have this problem, and many are traceable to early childhood and a reaction to the parents' demands. Here are some comments from one of my students:

"I was constantly late. My clocks were set some minutes fast so I could catch my bus to work on time. I had a tendency to start all my tasks at the last minute.

Carol took me back to one day before my birth. I remembered that my mother told me she had to postpone her studies at the college for one year because I was born. I arrived a week earlier than I was due and as a first child, I caused quite a stir. Apparently, I never wanted to be early again!

After the session with Carol, I am not procrastinating anymore. Now, I tend to start everything as soon as possible. I even set my clocks back to the proper time and I can catch my bus on time."

INDECISION

One of my interpreters asked me to help her with her indecisiveness. She could not trust herself to move forward in life, afraid that her decisions would be the wrong ones. We had to look at age three when her mother told her to cover her little baby brother, who was in a low cradle. So, she covered him completely including his head. She was punished for that and never wanted to take her own thought-out, direct action after that.

Because I worked with her often, it was interesting to watch her progress after our session. She said that of all her many stress release sessions during seminars and in private, this one was the most outstanding correction in her life, causing great changes.

We attended a wedding together near Budapest recently and she is still talking about it years later. What a difference a single session can make. Over the years, I have had the pleasure to watch her transform and grow into an even more beautiful person!

~

Following are three examples from a 29-year old student who volunteered for demonstrations in class. The topics cover fears, addictions and obsessions. We were quite amazed at how easily she put her stories together.

With each seminar, she volunteered and had incredible lessons for us. Since corrections for stress release done this way, openly, for other seminar attendees to observe, often benefit other members of the audience. We were also able to follow her progress from one seminar to another.

~

"Whenever I had to speak publicly, I began to cry. In the demonstration, we went back to age six when I had a conflict with my teacher, who was my own mother. As a student, she always felt I had to perform better than my peers. All my classmates were already out playing when I was still inside learning. I objected to that. At the age of six, I started to wear glasses because I could not see the blackboard properly. During the demonstration, I forgave my mother as I realized that she did what she did only for her daughter's sake. Now I do not cry for just any reason, I can read books easily, talk to my boss without stress, and I do not overburden myself anymore."

~

After a second demonstration she reported:

"I drank very little water. As a result, I had chronic inflammation in the pelvic area because of the kidneys. I withheld my urine and this is what led to the inflammation. I was very cautious and drank very little liquid all my life (as long as I could remember) so I would not have to urinate often.

In the seminar, we went back to age two when I had a problem with my grandmother. We lived in a village with no indoor plumbing. We had a metal potty which my grandmother used to put on the stove to warm in winter. One time the potty heated up too much and I burned my buttocks. It hurt for days, and I blamed my grandmother for that. (Two issues needed to be resolved, one minimizing water intake and the other, anger towards grandmother.)

After the session with Carol, I felt thirsty, drank more water at one time than I could ever recall, and I forgave my grandmother. All my previous, bad urine tests now have improved. I am no longer afraid to go to the toilet (before that, I drank very little in order to avoid going there). One week after the session, I perceived that both my kidneys were working properly again. I visited my grandmother's grave, put flowers on it and I felt very good forgiving her after 27 years."

~

This student's demonstrations continued with the issue of traveling:

"I had stress getting from one point to the other. We went back to six months before birth. At that time my mother took her university exams (during her pregnancy). Her husband could not be with her since he was in the army. My mother had great stress on traveling alone to have the baby.

Carol explained that the mother's stress hormones go through to the fetus. After the session with Carol, I got a new, much better job which involved traveling. I now have no problem with that. Prior to the session, I felt sick two days before I had to travel and I could not sleep, I also vomited many times. Now I enjoy my frequent travels with my new job!"

~

What a difference these sessions have made in the life of this young person. The joy she exudes is a pleasure for all of us to watch during our seminars together. She can now live a far different, happier, more peaceful life!

SLEEPING

When we cannot sleep well or wake up in the middle of the night and cannot get back to sleep, we must look at the emotional causes. Years ago I worked with a famous Hungarian actor. He would wake up at four each morning and start worrying about his career, which was very limited as was, therefore, his income. A month after his session with me, I picked up a magazine and his picture was on the cover. I have recently checked with him and he is very busy doing what he loves and is quite successful in his acting career.

~

Recently, at a party, I saw a one and a half-year old whose mother I had worked with earlier concerning the child's conception. Mom appeared overly weary. She reported that the child had been waking up as many as 16 times during the night since she was born. The mother would breast feed her several times during the night and then the child would sleep, but only briefly. We did a session on the child's stress going to four days before birth when this mother-to-be had a mother–in–law problem, the likely stressor, which we released. The mother was able to stop breast feeding baby during the night. From last report, baby is usually sleeping through the night.

SLEEP APNEA

This particular client had the type of sleep apnea where the breathing is temporarily interrupted during sleep because of a sinus blockage. She is also substantially overweight. She had gone into anaphylactic shock during sleep recently when she could not get her breath and had to be rushed to the hospital.

During this recent period, she had met someone after 17 years with whom she had not settled her stress. He was now working in the same office as she. My testing indicated that we had to look at age three where her family moved from the small village where she was the "star". All those wonderful caretakers (the whole village) suddenly disappeared from her life with the move.

In the new location, her other grandmother, who now helped to care for her, was a stranger. This client had not had a chance to understand and put closure on the earlier relationships and on the stress of the move from that tiny village. That lack of not putting closure on situations and relationships became a pattern in her life.

When her family did return to that village with her baby sister later, her sister became the "star" as the new, cute little baby. This client felt that the village was hers, not her sister's. During our session, we looked at many aspects of this problem including lack of closure, stress on moving (she has moved every ten years and feels compelled to move now) as well as becoming more "visible" with her excess weight problem. As our stress release session came to a conclusion, her breathing was much easier. She also felt much energy in her chest and flowing in her body. Now, she can take in the breath of life more fully.

~

When we are limited by many stressors in our life, it can affect our breathing physically as well as our mental and emotional approach to life. There is great symbology in our body and the conditions within it, as in the foregoing case. How do you feel when you are taking a deep relaxing breath on a wonderful sunny day: relieved, refreshed, renewed?

That breath is taking in our phenomenal gift of life. To breathe deeply is to take in the richness and fullness of life. To release the stress of the past and be relaxed in the present is our goal.

ADDICTION TO FAILURE

This gentleman's issue was that he loses because he can't manifest anything that has real value, especially financial. He is a Human Resources manager and good at this job, but his colleagues like to put everything on his shoulders. He starts something and then he gets disinterested. After a half year, he finds his jobs boring.

We went to age three with him. He recalled the happy times with his grandfather and eating freshly baked strudel. He remembered that his grandfather had a stroke and was taken away on a stretcher. As a tiny child he was very afraid of that situation. He was afraid when he went to visit his grandfather in the hospital and saw one side of his body paralyzed. His grandfather contracted pneumonia and died in the hospital. No one in the family expressed any emotion.

His father had a very bad childhood. In his adult life he worked with chemicals which caused his brain to shrink. He would have to lie in bed often for days, but then could go back to work for a while. When he wasn't feeling well, he became aggressive and would shout at them. During a robbery at his shop, he collapsed and died when my client was six. My client stated that when his grandfather died, his mother closed half down and when his father (her husband) passed, she closed down completely.

He was angry with her because she didn't feel capable, escaped reality and taught him to do the same. My client's mother had given up on any life's goals as well as on expressing emotion. She was just surviving. This was the example he was shown on how to manage life.

He had to forgive his mother and see life from her perspective. After releasing the stress from age three, my client said he felt as though he wanted to cry. He rarely ever cried--only when his mother died and again when he was cheated out of an award in school.

His new belief system is that one can be honest and manifest what he desires, not just survive like his mother, especially financially. He also learned that it is OK for him to express his emotions.

PROBLEMS OF THE TEENAGE YEARS:

ORIGINS OF OBSESSIONS

When we are obsessed with an object, person, place, thing, thought, habit, or substance, we have a fear that in the future we will not have enough of it. Therefore we can't enjoy what we have in the moment.

~

I had a student who was obsessed with cigarettes. He would hoard cartons of them and count them often. Daily he searched for the best prices and where to buy them. His whole world revolved around his preoccupation with his future concerning cigarettes. I have had the same observations with people obsessed with alcohol, gambling, hobbies, another person, and so on.

~

When we release the fears that were the underlying cause of addictions and obsessions, then we can be free to make other choices as to how we want to live our lives, free of limitations with which fears encase us. It is important to face all these obstacles, get them up on the conscious level, so we can deal with them. For instance, what is your problem with getting organized, following up, having enough time?

The following fears relative to your profession may cause addictions or obsessions to or about your work such as becoming a workaholic, perfectionist, making enough money, and so on. What are your addictions or obsessions in the following list? Do you have more to add than are listed here? How does stress on any of these affect you in present time or for the future? Too much or too little emphasis can be a result of fear from the past resulting in a compulsive behavior. Fear of:

1. Talking about your business to others
2. Belief in your business
3. Abundance
4. Bothering others
5. Responsibility
6. Leadership
7. Closing the deal
8. Being prejudice
9. Following-up
10. Rejection
11. Success
12. Failure
13. Certain expectations
14. The unknown
15. Commitment
16. Understanding the products/technology
17. Being worthy of profit
18. Being coach-able
19. Listening
20. Procrastination
21. Taking action
22. Asking questions
23. Managing time
24. Attracting the right people
25. Being positive
26. Being consistent
27. Attachment
28. Organization

Following is a testimonial of a 21-year old who came to me so distraught, saying that he did not have any reason to live! He was addicted to alcohol, drugs and cigarettes. I trust his story will help many young people having similar challenges, to know that there is a better, easier way to do life:

"I am a 25 year old French guy who wants to share the story of his life. It can be divided into three parts: the childhood travels, the teenage depression years, and the awakening.

I was born in Australia, because my parents happened to meet there, and I moved to China when I was two weeks old. At three years, I started kindergarten in Benin, West Africa. At six years I was home schooled in Albania and by eight, I experienced the first separation from my parents as I had to go to boarding school near Paris, on my own. When I was nine, my alcoholic father went to live in Zambia and my mother took me with her, first to Switzerland, then to Austria, where I graduated from high school.

Since the age of five, my deepest fear was that the ongoing struggle between my parents would finally result in my losing them. It became my reality. After the age of nine, I never ever again spent time with my father discussing life, poetry, literature, which used to make our relationship so special. I barely saw him one hour, once every two years and we had no other contact.

The relationship between my mother and me started to deteriorate, becoming an ongoing struggle as well, just as it had been between my parents. As a professionally busy mother that had to raise her teenager, I do know now that she did the best she could. However, back then, I could not forgive the pressure she was putting on me, her expectations that I could not meet, and the fact that she left my father, destroying the only thing that I cared for: my family.

The vicious cycle started: I was shy, didn't go towards others, so I felt rejected; but in fact I was excluding myself. My fears, my sadness, my lack of interest in living and my lack of interest in human beings in general, my growing hatred towards my mother led me to build myself a new identity. I decided to believe, when I was twelve, that drugs would be the only thing in life that can make me happy. That's how it became my world for almost ten more years. It was a wonderful world at the beginning, because you live extraordinary experiences where your body and mind are transported beyond their apparent limits. However, it is not possible to live happily that way. Addiction has a price which is enslavement and physical and psychological suffering.

I arrived in Budapest when I was 21, completely destroyed mentally. I didn't know who I was and how I could possibly get out of the pit I was in for ten years. Every little task seemed to require an enormous effort, like going out of the house or talking to people. I saw absolutely no other alternative than dying.

Until the day my path crossed the one of an angel, Carol, who introduced me to specialized kinesiology. I started to understand that you can blame the entire world and life for having hurt you, but in reality it will only reinforce your pain. Only you can make yourself happy and that is by loving yourself and others. If you integrate that in your daily life, you will be able to reach intense joy and inner peace within yourself, without any "external help" from substances of any kind.

But life has always surprises for you. As soon as I started to get better and the relationship between my mother and me improved tremendously, my father died at the age of 54 of throat cancer. It was a shock, but once you trust in life, you know deeply inside that everything that happens has its reason, and that it is useless to make yourself suffer because of reasons that are beyond your reach.

At the age of 23 I was diagnosed with cancer. I was exposed to the final test: Do you want to live or not? With the help of Carol's specialized kinesiology, I did react "unusually well" to the treatment according to my surgeon. I did refuse to be operated a second time, against the doctors advice, and I am perfectly healthy today.

Life will constantly test you, and you may have to face some difficult situations, but we all have the choice to make them painful, or not, by the way we react to them. Do you want to suffer and make your life difficult, or do you want to come out stronger and enjoy life? This can only be done by letting go of your fears and pain, your anger and resentment. If you don't see any solutions to your problems, know that there are angels out there ready to help you."

~

Note: This young man is living once again in Paris, has a part time job while back in university there and is in the top ranking in his class. He now has the skills and understanding (or may we say wisdom) to handle the many challenges that life offers for his growth, without being controlled by the fear and pain from his childhood.

ADDICTION TO COFFEE

If we need a substance in excess to feel good in present time, it is considered an addiction. One individual was addicted to coffee and to the odor which he said he found so wonderful. When we went to age five, he remembered having breakfast with his grandfather each morning. He loved his grandfather and wanted his approval. Therefore, he did just as his grandfather did. He soaked his bread in coffee so that he would get that smile of approval from grandpa.

He became addicted not only to the coffee but to looking outside himself for approval from others in practically all things that he undertook. For many years, he consumed more than six cups of coffee each day. Since our session, this person still enjoys the aroma of coffee, but is no longer addicted to drinking coffee.

AUTISM

There is a question of how to categorize autism. Because of my experience with it, I have decided to put it under compulsive behavior.

According to Wikepedia, "Autism is a brain development disorder that impairs social interaction and communication and causes restricted and repetitive behavior, all starting before a child is three years old. This set of signs distinguishes autism from milder autism spectrum disorders (ASD) such as Asperger syndrome.

Autism has a strong genetic basis, although the genetics of autism are complex and it is unclear whether ASD is explained more by multigene interactions or by rare mutations. In rare cases, autism is strongly associated with agents that cause birth defects. Other proposed causes, such as childhood vaccines, are controversial; the vaccine hypotheses lack convincing scientific evidence. Most recent reviews estimate a prevalence of one to two cases per 1,000 people for autism, and about six per 1,000 for ASD, with ASD averaging a 4.3:1 male-to-female ratio. The number of people known to have autism has increased dramatically since the 1980s, at least partly as a result of changes in diagnostic practice; the question of whether actual prevalence has increased is unresolved.

Autism affects many parts of the brain. How this occurs is poorly understood. Parents usually notice signs in the first two years of their child's life. Early behavioral or cognitive intervention can help children gain self-care, social, and communication skills. There is no known cure. Few children with autism live independently after reaching adulthood, but some become successful, and an autistic culture has developed, with some seeking a cure and others believing that autism is a condition rather than a disorder." (End of Wikipedia quote)

~

I will share two of my experiences with autism/Asperger syndrome. A few years ago I worked with a four-year old who was diagnosed with autism. He had a very short attention span, was extremely hyperactive and did not communicate in a normal manner. He could not be left alone. His parents were exhausted. After three sessions he showed amazing progress. Subsequently, a counselor at the special school he attended told the parents they would take care of him and they should not need to see me anymore. I have observed him as he grew older and now at age eight, he is nearly normal.

~

Very recently I worked with an eight-year old boy who was diagnosed with Asperger syndrome. When I observed him, he was hyperactive. He did not stop moving, made vocal noises constantly, lived in a dream world and had poor coordination. He is overweight, quite creative and very intelligent. He cannot make decisions. He requires an adult to sit beside him in school so he can be in a normal classroom.

The father related that recently, the six- and eight-year old sons were at camp together. They had a call from camp that the eight-year old had nearly strangled their six-year old apparently out of jealousy. His brother had just won an award for the outstanding camper of the week. The parents are unsure how to cope with this increasing challenge. He cannot be left unsupervised.

His father brought him to Budapest. He has so many deeply ingrained fears. He had such a great fear of flying, they had to force him to get on the plane. On the long plane ride (over nine hours, plus a six hour delay in take-off) he was sick to his stomach and had a dreadful trip. He was still very ill when we met them at their hotel the evening of their arrival.

In the first session, we worked on his current stomach ache and his condition in general. We found the most traumatic contributing factor was at age one and a half. When I asked his father what happened then, he said his new brother was born. When they brought the baby home from the hospital, the older brother collapsed upon seeing him. A new child in the home was apparently overwhelming. (A pediatrician once asked a mother to imagine how she would feel if her husband brought another woman home to live with them but said he would love and treat them both equally -- similar issue with siblings). We released the stress on this issue and talked about the relationship with his younger brother and how it could be better. Immediately after the session, he felt well so we went touring and to eat.

We next addressed his coordination. His father said that he cannot learn to ride a bike. He had worn out two sets of training wheels trying. His walking was demonstrably better after the session. His father had expected to spend the entire time with him doing very little but keeping him happy. The next day, they walked the entire day sightseeing in Budapest. He was busy drawing pictures of the castle, writing in his journal and identifying all the foreign cars. He had a great time, much to his father's surprise.

We worked on his decision making, with a major block at age two when apparently he made a decision that someone felt was wrong -- and let him know it. My final work with him was with his fear of flying. His father later told me that he had a very comfortable flight back home, enjoying the last sights of Budapest, staying awake the entire trip and seeing Cape Cod from the air. His changes have been impressive, but there is still work to be done such as detoxifying and changing his diet.

I recently had dinner with the family (in America) and I was amazed at his focus, calmness, communication and eye contact (previously missing). After my most recent work with him, his father reported that the next day he had an excellent email from his teacher on the child's positive change.

~

From my experiences in working with thousands of students and clients, I observed that when the energy is shut down in the meridian system, it can affect any part of the brain/body. The location in the body may depend on the emotion and where we may have an inherited weakness or deficiency. We must look at the emotions, and the physical contributors. With autism, I feel that there are so many insults to the emotional as well as the physical body of a baby or young child. The child programs into his thinking that the world is not a very nice place to be. He tunes out, especially to people who may cause him more pain! What physical insults come from our environment?

~

How we can get rid of much of the emotional and physical stress from the past and prevent future pain and fear, especially with our little children who depend upon us entirely for their safety and well being?

The jury is not in yet on such "dis-eases" as autism, but I have my own theory:

When growing up in the 1940s and 1950s, cancer was very rare, diseases such as Alzheimer's, Fibromyalgia, autism, Parkinson's, panic disorder, diabetes, obesity, hormone imbalances were not common. I do not believe it was because they were not diagnosed. Most of them just didn't exist. With modern technology, people are sicker than ever on the planet. What is the difference?

Now, our food is polluted and may have little nutritional value. Pesticides, insecticides, artificial fertilizers are destroying the nutrition of our plants. Hormones and antibiotics are in meat and dairy products. Our water is losing its vital life energy. Medications are being prescribed which have adverse side affects and fill the body with toxins. The air is filled with smog as well as the electrical waves from television, computers, cell phones, microwave ovens. That's the bad news! The good news is that we can take responsibility and clean up our acts and the environment. So many wonderful people have excellent creative ideas to overcome the challenges of our everyday living. We all have work to do! There are solutions.

CHAPTER 9

DYING AND DEATH

IN the human species at this time in our evolution, it seems that all of us will eventually confront these two topics. How we live our lives and how we feel about death and dying will determine how we face them. Our religious beliefs, as well as those of the society in which we live, and our experiences in life will shape our attitudes toward dying and death.

With rare exceptions, we all lose loved ones at some time. How well we adjust to this loss may be determined by how we feel about our own mortality. If we accept this as part of the human cycle, then our adjustments will be much easier.

Whether you believe in an after life or not, the main focus can be to have a good time here on earth while life lasts and do your best to live a life filled with good health, peace and love. It is not the years we live, but the quality of life while we live that is important. As a very young child, I had already come to realize that we are on earth to learn and to love. Of course, we all have our challenges, but that is how we learn. We can be grateful for the challenges and learn to handle them in the most effective way. That is what our work is all about --balancing life!

As Elizabeth Kubler-Ross pointed out, most people when dying say there are two regrets about their lives: they didn't tell someone they loved them and they didn't live out their life's dream. When asked what their life's dream was, they said they didn't know. How sadly incomplete!

As a very young child, I knew I wanted to help people and to be a teacher. All roads in my life led to that goal and it felt energizing when I was on track with it. My university degrees were in teaching. Then, my Montessori training was followed by my study of specialized kinesiology. With the latter, I knew I had found a methodology with which I could help our precious children (and adults).

Thus, I have dedicated my life to reaching as many people as possible in the world to impart to them the knowledge and wisdom I have gained since I began this special quest in 1980. When we live our dreams and have a fulfilled life, then at the end we can feel a special peace because we have completed our life's mission.

When I am working with a client on the death of a loved one, I ask them what they would like to say to that loved one if the deceased were present and what that loved one would say back to them. It is very healing for the grieving person to express in this way. It relieves so much stress. Perhaps they also need to work on a forgiveness issue, forgiving the departed or themselves for something that happened or didn't happen. I also ask them how that loved one would want them to feel now.

They need to realize that a grieving period is necessary, but they also need to get on with their lives, because their work here is not finished yet! So much healing of grief at the loss of a loved one can be accomplished in one session. When an individual can view the death and dying process more calmly, then they can accept their own mortality more easily. If we are not afraid to die, then we are not afraid to live more fully.

Following is my experience surrounding the passing of my 25-year old son, Robbie, from an inherited heart problem, hypertrophic cardiomyopathy. He left very unexpectedly and peacefully in his sleep. I am sharing this intimate information in the trust that it will help some parents and others to be comforted in their loss. One week before his passing, Robbie's last words to me were, "I love you, mom."

~

I happened to have been born into the Christian faith which has formed many of my belief systems. I believe in a loving God and also in an afterlife. These are my personal beliefs, but I respect the beliefs of all people.

I had written Robbie's eulogy, but asked a friend to read it for me because I didn't think I could. However, I could feel Robbie saying, "Mom, why don't you read my eulogy? I'll be right by your side and Grandma will be on the other side. You may shed a few tears, but not a lot." I delivered the eulogy with a calm composure, which I feel was possible only with their love and assistance. Many people at his memorial service said the eulogy was wonderful, that they had come to comfort me, but instead I comforted them. I felt I would mourn, but Robbie would not want me to grieve very long.

His sisters and I scattered part of his ashes at the canal among the beautiful nature he loved, and I scattered some in Prague, the city that he loved so much.

~

Several years ago, I received a book and CD order by mistake. I had asked Robbie to return it for me because I was returning to Budapest. He had it in his car for a while and then put it in his closet. When cleaning out his closet three days after his passing, I found it and opened it. In amazement I found that it was perfect for me at this time. There were eleven tiny booklets on how to deal with grief which I gave to our close family and friends, and two large grief books which I gave to his sisters. There were several CDs: The Tree of Life with the symbol of the Kabala (one of the greatest sources for truth which was recorded and kept pure knowledge alive during the Dark Ages). At the bottom of this CD was the name "Lauren" written in large letters, the name of Robbie's new niece. These CDs gave me great comfort during this period. There were two scarves imprinted with flying angels blowing horns. Among the several books was, "The Light Shall Set You Free". This is a very inspirational book dealing with esoteric information such as the Universal Laws. On page four was written, "Some books that none of us had ordered would appear mysteriously in the mail, providing precisely the reading material that was needed to help us gather information."

What kept Robbie from returning those books? On some deep level did he know how much comfort they would bring to me later? There was also a set of "The Game of Life Cards" (Affirmation and Inspirational cards). When his sisters and I scattered his ashes on the water, we each drew two cards. The messages were so appropriate for each of us. One of his sister's was, "Thy will be done this day! Today is the day of completion; I give thanks for this perfect day. Miracle shall follow miracle and wonders shall never cease." One of my cards read, "I cannot lose anything that belongs to me by Divine Right. I am under grace and not under law."

~

We have had so many co-incidences. A couple of months before his passing when I was visiting I said, "Robbie, remember when you used to hate the sound of the vacuum?" He said, "Yeah and I still do." When we were emptying and vacuuming his room, the vacuum shut off--then started itself again.

A few days after Robbie's passing I went to storage and of all the thousands of papers and records there, what should I come upon first, but two pages of his brilliant quotes from age five. Another coincidence?

There is a story that when someone departs, you will find pennies from heaven which is a message that they are fine. I find pennies, always old ones. Robbie didn't like shiny, new things. When I arrived in Prague, I began finding one koruna pieces, and in Budapest, one forint pieces. "One" is the symbol of new beginnings.

When he was taking violin lessons from ages three to seven years, the major work was done on variations of "Twinkle, Twinkle Little Star". Robbie listened to that tape each night for years and played it on his violin. Each night after bedtime stories and prayers, I usually played "Fur Elise" (one of Robbie's favorites) on the piano when we were living in Holland. I was visiting with a dear friend after Robbie's Memorial Service and her granddaughter's musical toy played both songs in succession! A little hello from Robbie?

When Robbie and his sister bought their home they shared, I had several prints from his favorite artists framed for them, including "The Starry Night". The framer covered a bit of one side, which Robbie noticed immediately and he commented on it. When I arrived back in Prague after his passing, on the wall of my hotel room...and then in my friend's kitchen was none other than: "The Starry Night"! He does have quite a sense of humor. A guilt trip for mom (because I had accepted an imperfect framing job)?

Robbie had been the most contented baby and child. He slept through the night at three weeks. But before that I would be up at night breast-feeding him while reading "The Thorn Birds". Recently I was attending the Budapest International Women's Club and spotted the "The Thorn Birds" novel at the very end of the used book table. I picked it up and read: "There is a legend about a bird which sings just once in its life, more sweetly than any creature on the face of the earth. From the moment it leaves the nest it searches for a thorn tree, and does not rest until it has found one. Then, singing among the savage branches, it impales itself upon the longest, sharpest spine. And, dying, it rises above its own agony to out-carol the lark and the nightingale. One superlative song, existence the price. But the whole world stills to listen and God in His heaven smiles. For the best is only bought at the cost of great pain... Or so says the legend."

Are all these events just coincidences? I think not. We don't understand very much about how God and the universe work!

ROBBIE'S EULOGY MAY 26, 2005

"A few weeks ago when I was visiting, I read what Robbie had written on the refrigerator magnetic pad:

"Truth is beauty, beauty truth.
That is all ye need to know on earth and all ye need to know."
From "Ode on a Grecian Urn" by John Keats

Robbie's life was about the search for the truth.

"Be ye not conformed to this world, but transformed to the next."
The conventional ways of this world were not Robbie's path to the truth.
Money, cars, possessions meant little to him. A car? He just needed
something to get around in. He spent many hours bike riding on a path
along the canal, enjoying nature in all its seasons.

Robbie had a voracious appetite for learning with a great passion
for the arts. At age two and one-half I can still see him riding his two-
wheel bike with training wheels beneath the fragrant plumeria blossoms
beside the coconut trees along our lawn in Venezuela. There at age two
he began his 12 years of Montessori Education, eventually spanning
three continents. This method fostered his individuality and deepened
his search for the truth. His focus and concentration were sharp from
an early age. At age three, his violin lessons gave him a deep apprecia-
tion of music, especially classical. Bach and Beethoven were his favorite
composers. He spent many hours at the piano trying to memorize Fur
Elise.

In Holland at the ripe old age of five, he conducted many tours for
our guests at the miniature village of Maduradam in The Hague. From
September to December he became fluent in Dutch in the Montessori
Preschool and became the family's official interpreter. Each winter day
after school (the canals froze that year just for us!), he and I would go to
the neighboring canal and ice skate.

In the summer, he was out enjoying nature with his sisters. He
would pull up his little lawn chair and sit for hours studying the ants
crawling in and out of the sidewalk cracks. On our ski trip to Austria, at
age five, he was instructing his Sunday school teacher how to snowplow.
Up to the highest mountain he would go with his sisters and come whiz-
zing down past us.

One of the highlights of living abroad was the vacationing with our
loving families; sharing peace, love and presents at Christmas, art and
swimming lessons with Nana, Easter Egg Hunts, fishing with Uncle Ta,
picking berries at Aunt Margaret's. These were precious and harmonious
times, which deeply enriched our lives.

His love of learning was in his time and in his way. He especially enjoyed the classics, and had an immense vocabulary. He amazed his family and friends with his vast trivia knowledge. When in the USA, I would ask, "Robbie, what would you like to do special?" He'd reply, "Let's go to Barnes and Noble." And off we'd go for a few hours. Can you imagine him now in the other perfect world with the Library of Alexandria, the Dead Sea Scrolls, and all the other great works of art, music, literature, and nature, perfectly intact?

His favorite spot in Prague was the James Joyce Irish Pub where the "intellectual" discussions of the day would take place. It came as no surprise that he named his three brother cats, Edgar, Allen and Poe.

Mundane details were not Robbie's forte. On one of his numerous trips to Europe, he attended a music seminar. His sister said, "Mom, you better check his passport." So I said, "Well, Robbie, when does your passport expire?" "Oh, yesterday." Off to the US Embassy and re-ticketing his flight we went! Now, to no longer need his passport where he is traveling, he must be elated!

Once, flying back to the USA together, he was delighted to be in first class and not have his knees around his ears. (He was 6' 5" tall.) He asked me for some paper and I thought he would write his impressions of this marvelous, magical, mystical city. Wrong! When I looked at his paper later, it was filled with mathematical formulas. On cereal boxes and all over the house, Robbie's formulas were etched. He engaged in teaching his college classmates calculus because his teachers had failed in the task. At a very early age he reached solutions without the process in mathematical problems.

I heard that he was a great dancer and entertained the whole disco in Budapest by dancing on stage. I thought this was a bit out of character for him.

Each time on my trips back he would have my favorite fresh whole-wheat, homemade bread ready for me. On my fourth visit this year, the bread was in the breadbox for me, but Robbie was on his new journey. He was a gourmet cook and it was a tradition for him to make Eggs Benedict for Christmas breakfast, over which his sisters always raved.

The greatest attribute of Robbie was his kind, gentle, loving, thoughtful manner. But the greatest of these was love, especially for his sisters, mother and father, his new niece, our extended family and friends. All who met Robbie loved him.

Thank you all for touching Robbie's life and our family's in a very special way. He takes that love with him on his soul's journey as he finds the truth in his now omnipotent, omniscient and omnipresent state. I am sure he is dignified by this celebration of his life and is enjoying his transition and the great peace and love in his new world. God bless you all."

~

Although the physical separation in death leaves a very deep void in our lives, I believe that we who are left behind are not finished here. We must continue on with the knowledge that our loved ones are in their perfect place and want us to be happy.

CHAPTER 10

FORGIVENESS, LOVE AND PEACE

WE may have heard the statement many times: "To forgive is Divine." But what does it really mean? We know what an impact our thoughts have on the body/mind as stated previously.

MRI scans prove how thinking of empathy and forgiveness can affect the brain. Fred Luskin, PhD, director of Stanford University's Forgiveness Project and author of "Forgive for Good" found that "letting go of negative emotions can cut your stress level up to 50 per cent while improving sleep quality, energy, mood and overall physical vitality".

When we let go of anger and are able to forgive, we stop the negative effects of the stress hormones relative to blood pressure, blood sugar, hardening of the arteries and countless other destructive functions. There is much more research which tells us that when we hold onto anger and resentment it has a toxic effect on the body because of the stress hormones that are released and not cleared out.

The body produces these stress hormones for an emergency situation and when the emergency is over, the body will rebalance. However, in our modern society, the adrenaline goes on for crisis number one of the day and before the body can rebalance we have crises number two, then three, then four… You get up in the morning already stressed because you are late, only to be greeted with the world's worst traffic jam. At work, you may have an unrealistic deadline, then you receive a call that your daughter is ill and must be taken home from school immediately, and so on. If we get upset with people and these situations and hold onto it, our body takes the punishment, sooner or later!

Stress is cumulative. How we <u>feel</u> about the problem is the <u>real</u> problem. How do we cope with pressure, unexpected and unwanted events and unpleasantly acting people? The key is in releasing the painful feeling in that memory, so it becomes just that, a memory. We must let go of the anger, fear, and frustration and forgive others whom we feel may have caused the situation. Then, it is necessary that we forgive ourselves for holding onto it.

If a child is abused by an adult, he will feel that there is something wrong with him, not with the adult. Thus, low self-esteem is programmed in and reinforced. So children who are sexually abused usually feel that it is their fault. The abusers know how to make these children feel guilty and use it against them. The child looks up to adults and trusts them. These feelings are recorded in the child's memory banks and patterns are set up in their continued behavior.

When an adult, he may intellectually look back and know the other adult was wrong, but those past beliefs are difficult to change unless we release the pain with that memory. Fortunately, the methods we use can erase this pain. The adult must learn to forgive that person from long ago. Howard Martin said, "Forgiveness releases you from the punishment of a self-made prison where you are both the inmate and the jailer."

First, it is important to understand that we, as individuals, and everyone else is doing the best they can. When we can see situations through the eyes of another's perception, then we have a better understanding of the whole, more of a worldview. At this juncture we can understand and have compassion and forgive. We all have our weaknesses because we are learning. We may not agree with another's viewpoint, but we need to be aware that they have their reasons for their views, beliefs, and behavioral patterns.

We do not condone such crimes as murder, rape or robberies, but we must understand why someone has behaved in that manner and not hold those negative emotions in our body.

Franklin P. Adams said, "To err is human, to forgive is infrequent." Why? Is it because we do not understand the positive results of that action: forgiveness. When we release those emotions of fear, anger and resentment, forgiveness can be very powerful. We can't change the past, but we can confront those unresolved issues and the stress on those people who contributed to those emotions. We don't even have to see them. Write a letter to them which you don't even have to send for it to be effective.

Remember this is all about <u>you</u> and getting the stress released from <u>you</u>! As a result of forgiving others and yourself, one can have a healthier, happier future! Believe me: it is worth the little energy it takes compared with all the energy you waste on all those negative feelings toward others and yourself! Write a letter to yourself. You don't have to send that one either.

The most important person and the most difficult person to forgive is yourself. How we love to punish ourselves! Look at your problems from many aspects. What led to that problem and what did you learn? Forgive your "self" and know that it was a valuable lesson. Thank your "self" for that lesson and live more wisely and abundantly.

~

In the following report, I saw this gentleman for two sessions. He was in the final phase of his battle with cancer. His big life issue, which he agreed to deal with, was forgiving certain members of his family with whom he had great stress.

I told my client the story of Nelson Mandela's forgiving. After Mandela's 27-year imprisonment, he invited his former jailers to his presidential inauguration. He was asked how he could do this, invite his jailers! He said that he knew that if he did not forgive them, he would be carrying his prison with him for the rest of his life! How many prisons do we carry with us that impede the energy flow in our bodies that eventually could possibly contribute to "dis-ease" in the body? It is not difficult to forgive.

After his first session my client made great progress in his forgiveness issue with his family members. His pain decreased, he was able to lower his pain medication, get on his tractor to mow his lawn, enjoy his horses, dogs and home. When he passed, even through the suffering, his soul was at peace. These are his words:

"CASE REPORT: I am a trauma surgeon."

"In 1999 I was diagnosed with cancer of the prostate (Gleeson # Seven) and underwent a radical prostatectomy. Thanks to my vigorous life style and basically good health, my recovery was rapid.

Five years later I began a series of escalating hormonal manipulation treatments directed by my oncologist for a gradually rising PSA. The treatments robbed me of my energy, caused a 50 pound weight gain, and were generally very debilitating. My doctor announced that my cancer was hormone insensitive and suggested chemotherapy which I refused.

Since the treatment was worse than the disease I elected to do nothing. I lost weight, was able to take care of my farm again and return to my more vigorous lifestyle.

In the summer of 2006 I developed a very painful boney metastasis in my spine which responded dramatically to localized radiation therapy. Things went well for a year until the summer of 2007 when I had a succession of boney metastasis in my spine and ribs which required multiple radiation treatments. These treatments became increasingly debilitating, although they did ameliorate the agonizing pain.

Within the last six months, pain control has become a major issue with gradually increasing doses of narcotics as I have reached my limits of radiation. I realized that my life as I knew it was being seriously compromised by my disease and drugs to the point where I was losing my will to live.

In May of 2008 I was hospitalized for a week to try to get my pain under control and more radiation. Results were not good; I was emotionally devastated and losing hope for any quality of lifestyle.

Being a zombie on narcotics for the pain is not a life. Carol Ann Hontz came to see me at my wife's request. She listened to my story and said "I can help you". She taught me several maneuvers for dealing with the pain and for the first time in five years offered me Hope. That simple act has had a profound effect on my attitude. My pain is currently under control and my major problem is withdrawal from drugs as well as the debilitating effects of so much radiation.

To have a hand held out with hope and a path towards restitution of my being, I am profoundly energized that I may have some good days left.

Thank you so much Carol Ann."

He did have some good days left to enjoy those things most dear to him. He wanted to go on a fishing trip in September. I wish him a good journey!

~

Forgiveness is paramount. The Buddha said, "Be kinder than necessary, for everyone you meet is fighting some kind of battle."

The following is a summary of some of the world's major religions on teaching forgiveness: "Forgiveness in Different Religions" from Deborah and Arvind's full Amazon blog.

BUDDHISM

Forgiveness is a practice for removing unhealthy emotions that would otherwise cause harm to our mental well-being. Hatred leaves a lasting effect on our karma and forgiveness creates emotions with a wholesome effect. Buddhism questions the reality of passions that give rise to anger through meditation and insight. After examination, we realize that anger is only an impermanent emotion that we can fully experience and then release.

Here are three Buddhist quotes on the folly of anger:

"Holding on to anger is like grasping a hot coal with the intent of throwing it at someone else but you are the one who gets burned"

— The Buddha

"You will not be punished for your anger. You will be punished by your anger."   — The Buddha

"It is natural for the immature to harm others. Getting angry with them is like resenting a fire for burning."   — Shantideva

SIKHISM

Forgiveness is viewed as the remedy to anger. You forgive an offender when aroused by compassion.

Compassion generates peace, tranquility, humility and co-operation in human interactions. The act of forgiveness is considered a divine gift, not the work of human agency. Otherwise, pride would increase when we take personal credit, which would impede our spiritual progress.

Anger is often considered the result of unfulfilled desire. If a person fulfills our desires and wants, we feel love for them but when they impede our desires anger can well up. The ego can easily feel slighted, embarrassed, belittled or in some other way be offended. As we learn to discipline our mind through meditation on the Word, our ego and anger naturally turn to compassion and forgiveness. Since anger and forgiveness are considered opposites, the human mind can only contain one of them at a given time.

Here are some verses from the Guru Granth Sahib, the Sikh scriptures, which capture the essence of forgiveness:

"To practice forgiveness is fasting, good conduct and contentment"
                                        — Guru Arjan Dev, page 223

"Where there is forgiveness, there God resides" — Kabir, page 137

"Dispelled is anger as forgiveness is grasped" –Guru Amar Das, page 233.

JUDAISM

Ideally a person who has caused harm, needs to sincerely apologize, then the wronged person is religiously bound to forgive. However, even without an apology, forgiveness is considered a pious act (Deot 6:9). *Teshuva* (, literally "Returning") is a way of atoning, which requires cessation of harmful act, regret over the act, confession and repentance. Yom Kippur is the Day of Atonement when Jews particularly strive to perform *teshuva*. Two relevant Jewish quotes on forgiveness:

"It is forbidden to be obdurate and not allow yourself to be appeased. On the contrary, one should be easily pacified and find it difficult to become angry. When asked by an offender for forgiveness, one should forgive with a sincere mind and a willing spirit."

— Mishneh Torah, *Teshuvah* 2:10

"Who takes vengeance or bears a grudge acts like one who, having cut one hand while handling a knife, avenges himself by stabbing the other hand."   — Jerusalem Talmud, Nedarim 9.4

CHRISTIANITY

In Christian teachings forgiveness of others plays an important role in spiritual life. The Lord's Prayer best exemplifies this attitude, notably in these words: "And forgive us our trespasses, as we forgive those who trespass against us" (Matthew 6:9-13). The final words uttered by Christ during his suffering reinforce the importance of forgiveness: ""Father, forgive them, for they know not what they do." (Luke 23:34). We also find instruction to love your enemies and turn the other cheek (Matthew 5:9 & Luke 6:27-31). Another beautiful expression of forgiveness and understanding is St. Francis of Assisi's prayer:

"Oh Divine Master, grant that I may not so much seek to be consoled as to console. To be understood as to understand. To be loved as to love. For it is in giving that we receive. It is in pardoning that we are pardoned. And it is in dying that we are born to eternal life. "

ISLAM

The word Islam is derived from the Semitic word "slm" meaning "peace". Forgiveness is a prerequisite for genuine peace. The Qur'an makes some allowance for violence but only to defend faith, property or life. Still forgiveness is held as the better course of action whenever possible: "They avoid gross sins and vice, and when angered they forgive." (Qur'an 42:37). In terms of clemency, we find this passage: "Although the just penalty for an injustice is an equivalent retribution, those who pardon and maintain righteousness are rewarded by God. He does not love the unjust" (Qur'an 42:40)."

When we forgive, we create a space for love in our hearts. Acceptance and love is the tie that binds humanity. It is the highest vibration. This love then creates peace.

THE GREATEST GIFT ... LOVE

It's time to tune up the strings of our instrument so that the masterpiece of life we now play is an exquisite one of great harmony and magnificence. It is our birthright. It was the way we were created to be.

In our rapidly changing world, we need to examine which old belief systems are no longer viable. We need to closely examine what solutions are producing positive changes for humankind. We need to get out of our old survival mode and thinking patterns and into the new options and choices. Drop what doesn't work.

In government, religion, education, business, commerce, technology there are wonderful people with creative, fresh new ideas who are providing us with stimulating leadership in a darkened world. Each of us needs to take personal responsibility for our own emotional healing. Only then will we have peace within and throughout the planet.

As I ponder the magnitude of the effects of our work with stress release, I always return to the essential emotion of the secret of living joyfully, vibrantly, creatively, productively, harmoniously, abundantly and peacefully. That emotion is love, and unconditionally loving yourself—NO MATTER WHAT!

If you perceive areas of your life where you need changes, recognize them, accept them -- and then make a plan to correct them. Secondly, when you love yourself unconditionally, you then have an amazing capacity to love others in the same way. You can understand where they are coming from and what their past programs are. Accept that and do not let it affect you. You may not choose to have a close relationship with them now if your belief systems are not similar, but you can still feel compassion and love for them.

Quite often I see where people have gotten rid of old behavioral patterns and belief systems which no longer serve them. Therefore, they leave close friendships or relationships whose way of acting on life no longer matches theirs. You move on to new, more meaningful relationships with greater sharing of ideas, values, work, hobbies, and central focus of life. You still love those friends -- but you may not be relating to them as fully as you did previously.

In stress release, we love each client unconditionally knowing that underneath that programming is a perfect, loving being. Love toward ourselves and others is the key. It creates harmony within, with others and throughout the earth. When we open our hearts to humanity, we are filled with compassion and wisdom.

We can learn to love without certain conditions. Love heals, creates peace within the soul. It gives us energy and revitalizes our spirit. Love is the greatest force to replace fear. Love is in a limitless supply. As love enshrouds us we feel tender and gentle. It brings us happiness, compassion and respect for all living creatures and respect for our planet. In closing, I wish to present a wonderful guide for living a full life.

The following is from Og Mandino's "The World's Greatest Salesman":

"I will greet this day with love in my heart, for this is the greatest secret of success in all ventures. A muscle can split a shield and even destroy life; but only the unseen powers of love can open the hearts of men. And until I master this art, I will remain no more than a peddler in the marketplace. I will make love my greatest weapon, and none on whom I call can defend against its force. My reasoning they may counter, my speech they may distrust, my apparel they may disapprove, my face they may reject and even my bargains may cause them suspicion; yet my love will melt all hearts. Like unto the sun whose rays soften the coldest clay I will greet this day with love in my heart.

And how will I do this? Henceforth I will look on all things with love and I will be born again. I will love the sun for it warms my bones. Yet I will love the rain for it cleanses my spirit. I will love the light for it shows me the way. Yet I will love the darkness for it shows me the stars. I will welcome happiness for it enlarges my heart. And I will endure sadness for it opens my soul. I will acknowledge rewards for they are my due. Yet will I welcome obstacles for they are my challenge.

I will greet this day with love in my heart. And how will I speak? I will laud my enemies and they will become friends. I will encourage my friends and they will become brothers. Always will I dig for reasons to applaud. Never will I scratch for excuses to gossip. When I am tempted to criticize, I will bite on my tongue. When I am moved to praise, I will shout from the roofs.

Is it not so that birds, the wind, the sea and all nature speak with the music of praise for their creator? Cannot I speak with the same music to his children? Henceforth, I will remember this secret and it will change my life. I will greet this day with love in my heart.

And how will I act? I will love all manner of men, for each has qualities to be admired even though they be hidden. With love I will tear down the wall of suspicion and hate which has built around their hearts and in its place will build bridges so that my love will enter their souls. I will love the ambitious for they can inspire me. I will love the failures for they can teach me. I will love the kings for they are but human. I will love the meek for they are divine. I will love the rich for they are yet lonely. I will love the poor for they are so many. I will love the young for the faith they hold. I will love the old for the wisdom they share. I will love the beautiful for their eyes of sadness. And I will love the ugly for their souls of peace. I will greet this day with love in my heart.

But how will I act to the actions of others? With love. For just as love is my weapon to open the hearts of men, love is also my shield to repulse the arrows of hate and the spears of anger. Adversity and discouragement will beat against my new shield and become as the softest of rains. My shield will protect me in the marketplace and sustain me when I am alone. It will uplift me in moments of despair; yet it will calm me in times of exultation. It will become stronger and more protective with use until one day I will cast it aside and walk unencumbered among all manner of men, and when I do my name will be raised high on the pyramid of life. I will greet this day with love in my heart.

And how will I confront each who I meet? In only one way, in silence and to myself. I will address him and say, "I love you". Though spoken in silence these words will shine in my eyes, un-wrinkle my brow, bring a smile to my lips, an echo to my voice and his heart will be opened. And who is there who will say nay to my goods when his heart feels my love?

I will greet this day with love in my heart and most of all I will love myself. For when I do I will zealously inspect all things which enter my body, my mind, my soul and my heart. Never will I over-indulge the requests of my flesh. Rather I will cherish my body with cleanliness and moderation. Never will I allow my mind to be attracted to evil and despair. Rather I will uplift it with the knowledge of the ages. Never will I allow my soul to become complacent and satisfied. Rather I will feed it with meditation and prayer. Never will I allow my heart to become small and bitter. Rather I will share it and it will grow and warm the earth. I will greet this day with love in my heart.

Henceforth I will love all mankind. From this moment all hate is let from my veins. For I have not time to hate; I have only time to love. From this moment I take the first step required to become a man among men. With love I will increase my service one hundred fold and become a great co-server. I have no other qualities I can succeed with love alone. Without it, I will fail though I possess all the knowledge and skills of the world. I will greet this day with love and I will succeed."

With forgiveness and love as your foundation, you may truly say:

HELLO HAPPINESS!

Letters From Students

Following are some comments from students of my recent Metamorphosis Series:

"Dear Carol,

Thank you so much for providing us with such a lovely, informative and *transformative* weekend. I've been spending what I think is nothing less than *every free second I have* using the techniques you taught me on myself for so many wonderful corrections. I've also used it on several occasions with friends and clients - with some great results. I've found it to be such a monumental and expeditious form of healing ... I am just so grateful that Laurel and Carol sent me the note about you - and I've already started spreading the word for your seminar and appointments in the future.

I am a changed and lighter woman, as you could already see after the first day of the workshop, and I am so grateful you are sharing these wonderful techniques in such a relaxed, fun, loving, accepting, and easy to understand format. I'm so grateful for every piece of the experience, not the least of which is getting to know your wonderful soul as well as the kind souls of the others at the workshop.

What a complete gift! Thank you so much for blessing my life. Love and Light to you, A. "

~

"Dear Carol,

What a lovely title for your soon to debut book. I am including your workshops I've attended in my school contract for the summer so my bachelor's degree can come to fruition. I would appreciate a paragraph from you verifying and perhaps saluting my presence in your courses. My gratefulness for your courses can be seen in the contentment I am experiencing in my life and the lives of friends and family.

The work is profound and ripples out lifting the vibrations and eluci-
dating that which would otherwise go unseen. Basically in the slang
of my contemporaries-- You Rule! You Rock! The work you've culled
and employ is changing the structural architecture of every aspect of
the way my existence co-exists with humans, animals, plants and the
like." "S."

~

"Dear Kathleen,

I wanted to thank you so much for bringing Carol Hontz to Baltimore
this past fall. She is an amazing person, like you, and I will never
forget the wise strength exuding from her soft, loving eyes when she
spoke to me in front of all the workshop participants and friends.
She said, "So with all the times you've been rejected, what's one more
time?!" I used that memory-moment to help me complete my recent
award in my company, whenever I felt afraid to ask for the appointment or the sale!

The other "Ah-Ha" moments were watching the transformation of
others she worked with, seeing them change their limiting beliefs
(often habitual and life-long negative beliefs!) right before our eyes!

On a personal level, in my private session with her, we discovered some
tragic moments in my life that had me continually beating myself up
over and feel "unworthy". Carol gently led me to feel forgiveness and
compassion for myself and others, back to a state of grace.

Of course, being human, there will always be "dragons to slay", but
when I was first introduced to Carol through you, I had had an accident and was in a very dark place—so you asked her to help me and I
am forever grateful to you both. As she pulled her energy-magic "out
of the hat" (and worked with me all the way from Budapest), I truly
felt some of my anguish release! Now, the dark memory has no hold
on me.

I cannot wait to continue working with her techniques to help unleash my unlimited potential!"

'L." January, 2008

~

"I had the good fortune of attending Carol Ann Hontz' workshop "Can We Talk" in Baltimore hosted by Kathleen. I had no idea what to expect, but I was open to whatever experience presented itself. What happened over the next two days was unexpected, unbelievable and wonderful.

First let me say that Carol Ann's aura is charismatic. There is such a sense of serenity and peace combined with an air of enjoyment and excitement in her delivery of the subject matter that the positive energy is contagious. The audience is compelled to listen and learn whether they want to or not.

Over the course of the workshop, the audience was repeatedly moved witnessing the wonders of watching people who broke through the weight of carrying lifelong burdens they had heretofore harbored, in many cases unknowingly, that had negatively affected their actions, behavior, thoughts, business decisions, progress, success and more. The breakthroughs were palpable and visible to all. We watched mesmerized at the transformation as each person's entire demeanor changed as the stress lifted, replaced with tranquility and confidence.

The primary purpose of the workshop was to address public speaking phobias, but I am convinced that everybody who attended the two days got so much more out of it on both a personal and professional level. In fact, I would venture to say that after the workshop, everybody's productivity and satisfaction in their personal and business life increased exponentially. As a business owner, it is my intention that as soon as I have a sufficient amount of employees, I will insist that everybody attend one of Carol Ann Hontz' workshops because I see a huge benefit professionally and personally to opening the door for everybody to experience the possibility of living to their true potential. In the big picture, if people feel good and believe in themselves, then we all benefit with a win/win situation. Isn't that what it is all about?

My sincerest thanks to Kathleen for having the insight and open mindedness to take a huge leap of faith and give her people a gift that has lifelong ramifications in the most positive way.

"B."

ALL THE BROKEN HORSES
(A STUDENT'S STORY)

"We don't have the money to spend on knick-knacks. If you can find a broken horse, maybe someone will give it to you," my father says. My young inner self hears, "You aren't worth the price of a whole, undamaged china horse. You are only worth the free, discarded, broken ones." My inner translator stamps on my brain, "You are only worth what no one else wants. You are not worthy of great stuff. You are lucky to get leftovers."

Later in Life: Teachers are workhorses. They are always "in the harness". New teachers are "champing at the bit" to get started. You "get back in the saddle" after being gone. You "take up the reins" each new school year.

Still Later: When you retire, you are "put out to pasture" like a worthless horse that no one can use any more but haven't the heart to kill. So—you are not only worthless, you are unwanted and undeserving of good.

MEMORY
(THE STUDENT'S STORY CONTINUED)

"You've been bad—no ice cream for you! You are WRONG—go to your room and don't come out until you say you're WRONG!" my father orders. (But I'm NOT wrong.)

"Yum-m-m-m-! We're having ice cream and you can have it if you say you're WRONG!" (That would be a lie—I'm not wrong.)

"SAY YOU'RE WRONG!"

(I don't get ice cream very often—but saying I'm wrong would make me a liar. I did no wrong. So I sit in a dark room listening to my family eating ice cream—and I cry.)

Born in the early 50's to a controlling father and a now cowed and submissive mother, my life was one of near poverty and abuse. My father ruled us totally. He decided what kinds of used clothes we could take from the missionary barrel to wear, what hairstyle we were allowed, what books we read. He ate the best and his fill of what we had and his will was ours, or it had better be if you wanted to avoid a beating with the leather belt he hung in the closet.

At a young age, I saw discrepancies in his teachings, but when I questioned them, I was "of the devil" and was beaten. I was also "cursed" with intuition, but learned to keep that quiet for survival sake.

Although I was the first grandchild on either side of the family, I was a girl. When my brother was born, I was "discarded" emotionally and ignored in favor of the "blessed" male. He was what mattered, not a mere female, so I tried throughout my life to be better, faster, and smarter than the male population so I could receive some sort of recognition.

When the sexual abuse started, I also longed unconsciously to be male. Maybe "he" (my father) wouldn't do those things if I were a boy. I began to gain weight—in an unconscious attempt to become unattractive. Men don't like fat women. If he didn't like me, maybe he would leave me alone. No such luck. Although he was obsessed with looking young and trim, the abuse continued. If I did not submit, he would do it to my younger sister, he said. I was already "damaged goods". Maybe I could save her. Later I discovered I had not. He had abused her as well, although not as severely. He also later abused my nieces (his grandchildren) and had made attempts (some successful??) on various women ... during counseling sessions. When confronted by others, concerning one woman who came forward and accused him, my father convinced them she was having fantasies about him and her whole family was expelled from the church. To the outer world, he presented the façade of a caring man of God. Only our family saw his true self.

My mother died when I was 24 and my father remarried. My siblings grew, married and started lives of their own. Throughout my adult life, I tried to undo the conditioning of my youth. I began to follow my own spiritual path and to embrace my "other world" gifts. My abilities were revealed to few and to none of my family. I learned shamanic journeying and soul retrieval, became a Reiki master in five traditions and studied many religions and spiritual teachings in an effort to understand what my soul sought. Who was I and why was I here? I began to write what my soul wanted to say, to draw what my inner eyes saw. Still, I shared the results with few. Afraid, the inner child was afraid.

Years passed and I retired from teaching school. Releasing most of my belongings, I moved across country. New friends, new places, but abundance still just beyond my reach. My pension did not quite cover basics and so I did substitute teaching, designed jewelry, did clay work and drew, all trying to make ends meet and have a bit extra so I could continue to do the jewelry design and clay work I love so much. And I wrote—poems, short stories, three novella length stories. Studying, working, peeling away at the onion layers of my life—but it was going so very slowly.

A friend told me of a specialized kinesiology teacher she had studied with and was going to see again. Interesting, but I had no money to pursue it. A few months later, the same friend emailed me that the same teacher, Carol Ann Hontz, was going to present seminars in a nearby town. I replied, asking what changes my friend had experienced. I was impressed with her answer. Maybe this was something I should look into?

An email flyer arrived, telling about the seminars, personal sessions and a free lecture. I read and reread the information. Money was very tight. It was end of summer and I hadn't had a substitute teaching paycheck since June. I sat and stared at the picture of Carol Ann and somehow KNEW she could help, that I would be safe, that I had to do this. In a leap of faith, I scheduled a personal session and signed up for one seminar. My friend had scheduled a personal session right after mine, so we carpooled, planning to stay for the free lecture as well.

Carol Ann's method was so gentle and yet went deep into the mind of my inner child. Blocks shattered. I slept on a couch while my friend had her session. During Carol Ann's lecture, I was chosen for one of the demonstration clearings. A fear of high open places that I have had for most of my life was released.

As I listened to her information and real life examples, I knew I needed another seminar of the ones she offered the next week. Another leap of faith. It would take all but $15 of my money to pay for it. I told no one. The inner child was afraid. The adult me said—TRUST.

Four days of seminars. Like someone stranded in the dessert being offered water, I drank. My soul filled as the layers of conditioning fell gently away. Insights came. Light returned—light that had been extinguished at birth.

One final seminar remained—one I wanted, needed to take. But the money was gone. Carol Ann came around and asked each of us if we were coming to the final class. I confided my situation and, graciously, she said we could work something out.

On the drive back home, I realized I had no money, BUT I did have jewelry—one-of-a-kind items I had created—that I could offer. With hope in my heart, I gathered several pieces I thought would appeal to Carol Ann and brought them with me the next day. I was not only able to trade for the price of the seminar, but also sold pieces to other participants as well. I received back most of the money I had trustingly spent on the classes. Guess what seminar I just finished? ABUNDANCE! It works!

I am so grateful to Carol Ann for developing this powerful yet gentle method. I am grateful for her patience and willingness to share this with us. She is truly a light in the darkness. Thanks to her, the layers of my onion are much fewer and I am looking forward to taking more classes in the future."

--(any form of identification withheld by request.)

Note: One of my clients admired the necklace made by this person and said she could sell many of them, so I put them in touch. Abundance is continuing!

~

"Dear Carol Ann,

Since meeting you I have accomplished things that I never thought were possible for me. I think it's time to give you the testimonial I have promised you for so long.

Carol Ann Hontz calls her brand of "specialized kinesiology" Metamorphosis. I want to tell you that the name Metamorphosis is a perfect choice for the transformation that takes place after you receive a session from Carol Ann.

After attending two of her workshops and seeing her for two private sessions I became aware that I was a caterpillar inching my way along life's path. But in one short year I am now an iridescent butterfly spreading her wings and flying toward the life I was meant to live. Carol Ann worked with me on my eyesight and dyslexia. As the caterpillar, I was blind to things I needed to see from my past that were holding me back. Now my dyslexia is 99% gone and I can see and sense things as a butterfly that leads me to the sweet things in life. My past traumas are released as I continue to release them from my new view. Carol worked with me in the "Mental Sharpening" workshop and we discovered that I had a hearing imbalance. She took me back to 3 days before I was born. What wasn't I able to hear? It was that my birthmother was deeply saddened about having to give me up for adoption. My hearing improved as soon as I found the adoptee support group that I now attend. It is preparing me emotionally as I actively search for my birthmother. I had always been afraid to search for her, so I hid in a chrysalis, blind and deaf to my need to know who I am and where I came from.

With my newfound freedom I have been able to do things I never thought were possible like using Carol Ann's kinesiology in my CranioSacral light touch therapy work. I took Carol Ann's "Can We Talk" workshop in Baltimore and am now putting together a demo for my practice. Just a week ago I gave an intro speech for a colleague of mine at a business luncheon and I had so much fun using what I had learned from Carol Ann. I used to dread those situations. Now I can't wait to give my own speeches. If something is holding you back you release it and sooner rather than later, it is gone because you have released the energy blockage that was holding the traumatic pattern in your body.

The last example I want to share is so important because it connects Carol Ann's work to all of us here in the USA and the world at large. With my newfound courage to fly and try things I had never done, I signed up to campaign for Barack Obama. I met and telephoned many people from both the left, right, and in between. It was really difficult talking to the people who were so afraid and angry. Of course Carol Ann's commitment to the being in love and light helped me connect to the most positive energy so I was able to speak to everyone with the calm that is embodied by Barack Obama. I do believe that if it were not for the bringers of Light like Carol Ann Hontz the election could have gone in the other direction. I am so glad we chose Hope and not Fear.

As Carol Ann says we have the opportunity to chose once we learn how to let go of the stress. So listen to the butterfly who lived in the dark for way too long. Break out of your cocoon and get to one of Carol Ann's workshops ASAP. You will be happy you did. Bring a friend and share the fun!

Carol Ann, you know how much I respect and love the work you so lovingly share with all of us." "S"

METAMORPHOSIS SEMINARS

Following is a description of the "Metamorphosis" Seminars which I have created, based on my thousands of hours of study in numerous areas of specialized kinesiology and 28 years of experience with it. They are easy to learn and very effective. I have created them as two-day courses which can be taken in any order after the first basic course. We are so busy in our lives, I wanted to create a system that could give students maximum benefit in a short time with little expense.

MENTAL SHARPENING

Remove blocks to being sharp and aware, using your fuller potential, fuller mental acuity, eliminating stress. This course, a preferred prerequisite, teaches basic techniques which will be used in all the other courses.

Want to change your life? Change your belief systems and patterns. We invite you to attend this two-day seminar where you can learn effective techniques and get educational insights to cancel the fear and pain of the past and reconnect the body, mind and spirit. Take back your power and shed any destructive belief systems. Become who you really are! Specialized kinesiology (bio-feedback) is very gentle, non-invasive and an effective way of getting rid of the root cause of fears, allergies, pain, learning problems, all sorts of mental, physical and emotional problems. It is especially effective with learning and problem solving. In this course we will focus on releasing the fear and pain of the past which has affected our ability to learn easily. A sharp mind makes for a happy, productive, creative, healthy and abundant life.

Stress on reading, writing, hearing, speaking, mathematics, linguistics, vision, and life, will be addressed in this comprehensive course.

We welcome all for an exciting adventure into opening more of your great potential!

EVOLVING RELATIONSHIPS

Relationships, it's the number one stressor of the times. How are your primary relationships, relationships with your colleagues, your boss, your employees, your parents, your children, your mother-in-law, your friends, your neighbors? Are we into separation and no-choice in those relationships, repeating the same behavioral patterns of control or being controlled for a lifetime? Can we change those self-destructive patterns that are based on our fear and pain from the past? Through stress release we are able to break down the limitations that block us in developing healthy relationships. Through awareness we are able to create the kinds of relationships we desire.

However, we must keep in mind the most important relationship is with ourselves. With acceptance of self we gain the high esteem that is necessary in the development of our infinite potential.

In this seminar, we will take a fresh approach to the reason we are in relationships and what we have to do and learn within those circumstances. We shall stress release the root causes within ourselves for the negative responses and actions we manifest in relationships. With clarity and choice, we can then choose different constructive responses and actions. Bring peace, harmony and understanding into those troubled relationships!

BALANCING THE BODY

Balance is the key to harmonized living. Too much or too little of anything which our body, mind and spirit need to sustain life, creates imbalance and will make us ill. Anything our body does not need, such as toxins, electro-magnetic smog, etc., will make us ill. According to Webster's dictionary, "nutriment" is something that nourishes or promotes growth, provides energy, repairs body tissue and maintains life. What components accomplish these goals in life?

In our modern day world, how can we achieve balance in our bodies, minds, emotions and spirits? The answers lie in educating ourselves and our families on how to clean up our lives!

This two-day seminar is designed to provide updated research on the causes for so many of our modern day dis-eases and to show how to balance our energy so that we can maintain our bodies at a high energy level. Imbalances may be caused by toxins in the home and outer environment, synthetic hormones and drugs, diet and nutritional deficiencies, lifestyles and belief systems. These areas will be addressed with solutions using some effective, inexpensive, and efficient alternatives for living a healthy life.

The seminar will offer techniques to balance the physical body through the emotions as well as information on testing food, detoxifying safely and creating and living a healthy lifestyle, in spite of what is happening in the outside environment.

ABUNDANCE

When we think of abundance today, our main emphasis is on money. However there is a much broader approach to abundance in all areas of life. If we have low self-esteem, then we may not believe that we deserve the best in life, including the money we desire. Money is energy. Isn't it interesting that we came into life without money on our person, we will go out of life without it, but still it is the chief concern of a majority of people?

What belief systems do you hold about money? Could it be in the lack of understanding of the principles of abundance? Could it have to do with self-worth, with what is good and what is evil? How often have you heard or said: money is the root of all evil, money corrupts, money doesn't grow on trees, money is scarce, and money is never freely given. We may have the basic belief that there is never enough...of everything, not just money!

In this seminar you will have an opportunity to empty your mind of those old thoughts that were programmed in long ago. We will release blocks on all areas of life where we would like abundance: relationships, health, careers, etc. (not only financial). Failure is due to failure-thinking. Poverty leads to all kinds of crime, family problems, alcoholism, drugs, tension, stress and other health problems. Let's clean up our thoughts! Choose an abundant life!

TIME

In this seminar we will remove blocks relating to our concept of time and how we use time. To live in the "now" moment is key to expressing our true self and nature. We have a thought and later the creation.

When we control our thoughts concerning time we can create the future that we want. What we feel and think about past events traps us in the past. We become one with life when we eliminate the stress from the past and worry about the future. Then we can live in the "now" breaking through the illusion of time. When we identify with and are addicted to the whims of the ego, possessions, events, thoughts, emotions, we are buying into the illusion of time.

Happiness is wrongly focused on having, being and doing more, which takes us out of present time, since the yearning for more means that we are never really satisfied. With less ego reaction, we are empowered and do not waste our precious energy and time.

Young children know how to live in the "now" and practice the magic of no time. They do not worry about what happened yesterday or about what will happen tomorrow.

For everything there is a season...Come learn how to work efficiently and effectively with the illusion of time, respecting the windows of time allotted to us to complete our missions on this earth journey.

SLIM, TRIM AND FIT

The United States has the highest obesity rates in the world, with 67 per cent of the adults and children overweight, according to "Time" magazine of December 1, 2008. Other nations are rapidly following the American pattern. Fast food and lack of exercise contribute greatly to this trend. The growth of the fast food chains has made high-fat, inexpensive meals readily available. How are the eating habits of children programmed? The tastes that a child develops in childhood are retained into adulthood. They develop a taste for fats and sugar at a very early age, especially in baby food and drinks. A European Union study showed that 95 per cent of the food advertising for children encouraged children to eat foods high in sugar, salt and fat.

What is the cost to individuals and society? Obese people suffer from low self-esteem and emotional pain. Obese American children are dying from heart attacks and other related diseases. Obesity is a major killer in the USA. American health care costs are in the hundred of billions of dollars annually for obesity. It was recently estimated that nearly 300,000 Americans die every year because of the results of being overweight.

In this seminar, the emotional cause of our attitudes and actions with food (including the conditions of anorexia and bulimia) are examined and negative emotions released. Learn how to take responsibility for your eating habits; it's an inside job! Learn how to behave in front of food!

CAN WE TALK?

You can, if you think you can, fulfill your speaking potential. Fear of public speaking is one of the greatest fears in the world today. From where did it come? How can we be rid of it? Most of us were not born with the fear of public speaking; we acquired it. This fear is not really a part of us, so we can remove it as we would a piece of clothing. As tiny babies, we expressed openly and freely. We cooed, laughed, cried; we didn't care who was listening…that is, until someone gave us the message that it was not correct, through their comments, body language or punishments. The deep subconscious programs are planted very early in the brain/body with each subsequent negative experience layering over to create a deeper degree of fear.

How many times in school were we criticized, or even chastised, when we said something "they" considered wrong? Our thoughts have the power to control our physical and mental actions so that we are reacting out of the fear and pain of the past many times. We are able to access that memory which was stressful long ago and restore the body/brain to its normal neurological flow.

This seminar focuses on getting rid of the fear and pain of the past which the individual had locked into the brain/body. It also focuses on releasing the blocks associated with skills to becoming a better speaker. You can if you think and feel you can!

SELF ESTEEM

Are you being true to yourself or have you become other people's expectations? Do you feel responsible to make other people happy, even if it makes you feel badly? What is your self-talk about? Do you praise yourself or downgrade yourself? Do you praise others and are you happy for their success? Are you just playing a role and acting out a part in life that is not really the wonderful person you were created to be? Are you identifying with your profession? What happens when you retire from that profession? Are you then a nobody?

You are a unique, expressing human being unlike anyone else on the planet. No one else has your genes, your life experience, talents, wisdom, and skills.

When we are quiet, the answers and solutions come and show us how to accomplish our goals. The right people and circumstances will come to us.

You are not really the roles you are playing. If you are feeling inferior and incomplete, then you are not living up to your full potential. In this state you will feel exhausted and depleted of vital energy because you are not the real you that you were created to be. This seminar will remove the blocks for you to discover who you are and what you should be doing with your life. Come enjoy the banquet of life!

WELLNESS, OUR NATURAL STATE

Our natural state is perfect health, happiness and abundance, but we forgot how to keep and re-create this state. As tiny babies, most of us had perfect health. What happened between then and now? When our emotions are in balance, our bodies will follow. Then the harmony within begins to externalize and our lives and our environment are transformed.

In our daily routines there is much opportunity to feel and express harmony. If we continually repeat the same old patterns, then the growth does not come and we waste much time and energy. If we think and work constructively and in joy, it will enrich our lives.

It is ironic how carefully we guard our possessions, but allow the most precious possession of all, our inner peace, to be destroyed by challenges and fear. When we take back our power, we realize there is nothing that can throw us off balance.

For creating inner harmony and to use our energy constructively, we must let go of the fear and pain from the past that limits us and take our place in the world. Focus on positive thinking and acting, and you will have more beauty, love, perfection and abundance in your life.

Learn what changes you can make to balance your inside and outside worlds to give you vibrant health, and power. Get back your birthright!

TARGET THE GOAL

What is success? Success is not only wealth, but it can also be in relationships, good health, creativity, security and peace of mind. When we get in touch with our creative potential and express it, our life goals can be reached effortlessly. We have so much unrealized power within each of us. Because of our fear-based idea of limitation, we withhold our expression. We worry about what others will think or say, judging ourselves and others, which takes energy.

We are each part of a universal energy field that has pure potential. We can reach out, grab a handful of unformed energy and mold it into what we want. That is actually what we do! Bill Gates lives in the same energy field as you do and uses the same potential energy to which you also have access to! Look what he has done with some of it! There is a lot more waiting for you!

When we are quiet, the answers and solutions come and show us how to accomplish our goals. The right people and the right circumstances will come to us.

In this seminar we will rid you of some of those limited thinking patterns: fear-based limitation, judgments, and control issues. Then you can enjoy the freedom to express and feel life flow with ease and joy, delighted to be alive to achieve your mission here in the world! Come enjoy the banquet of life!

BUSINESS WITH INTEGRITY

We are graduating to a world where we realize that we are all one. The globe is shrinking, we all must breathe the same air, drink the same water and eat from the same food sources. We are all interconnected by our mobile phones and internet. What does this mean in terms of the business world? The success of one individual affects us all. A win/win approach demands that we have direct, open, honest communication and celebrate everyone's success as well as our own. In this course, we remove the blocks of jealousy, greed and competition so we may be the best person we can be for ourselves. When we are on our mission, then it is good for everyone. Then we can be on our place in the world, where no one else can be.

The purpose of this seminar is to give you the opportunity to further examine your belief systems about business, money, personal and professional relationships, consideration of the environment, with a major emphasis on self- esteem and integrity. There are universal principles which govern us and apply to everyone, everywhere, all the time. If we are in harmony with those principles in our interactions with all people, places and things, then our business will flow smoothly, as well as our lives. Business and our business of living are inseparable.

CONFLICT RESOLUTION

Conflict is usually very emotional. Instead of attacking the other person, we must attack the problem. What are the causes(not the symptoms)? What lies behind the emotions? Resentment and anger do not solve the conflict. When we are not reacting out of fear from the past, we can see other options clearly. It is important to act immediately so we do not lose an opportunity when the conflict is fresh and current. It is important to listen actively to the other parties involved. Consider the intonation and body language. Deal with all aspects fairly to the best interests of all concerned. There is always a best solution for all involved. Be clear within yourself. Express your own needs and concerns and tell how you feel, what it is you want in this situation and what you are willing to do to get that. Be clear and non-threatening.

In this seminar we will release the blockages that are keeping us from seeing the problem clearly, communicating effectively, listening, looking beyond the emotions, seeing other options, forgiving, discussing the problem in the moment as it comes up for discussion, accepting responsibility, and seeing a positive solution for the future.

Come find out how to resolve conflicts without hurting yourself or the other side and how to have peace in that situation and in future situations in your life.

FEARS = ADDICTIONS = OBSESSIONS

Only a decision is required to change one's mind. How do we reach a decision to change our minds about a conditioned fear of which we may not even recognize the origins? Fear affects all areas of our lives: personally and professionally. If we do not handle the fears of our early childhood, they will be manifested later as our addictions, keeping us feeling good in present time and suppressing the fears of the past. Alcohol and drugs are a perfect example of how we do this. If we do not handle the present time addictions they become our obsessions for the future, for example: not being clean enough, having enough alcohol and drugs for the future. The obsessed individual may constantly be counting his bottles of alcohol or cigarette packages.

Fears attach themselves to us like barnacles. They are not really a part of us, but just a belief system which we have acquired because of our feelings about a past traumatic situation. It is held in the body by thought and by the attention we give it. The more times one says s/he is afraid of spiders, the deeper ingrained the fear, the greater the fear reaction to spiders. If you are afraid of spiders and you talk about it, all the spiders available will find you!

This seminar will help to rid you of your major fears that are limiting you both professionally and personally as well as releasing your major addictions and obsessions.

EDUCATION AND SOCIAL RESPONSIBILITY

Much emotional damage is done to very young children. Parents and teachers need to understand the true nature of the child. Very early in life, we were expected to perform in a certain way to meet others expectations, whether we wanted to or were even capable of reaching their standards set for us. If we did not, we thought there was something wrong with us and down went the self-esteem and we become others' expectations to survive.

What is the purpose of education in our societies? Is it only to pass on facts or is it to acquire tools for living a harmonious life in wisdom. What can we conclude about our past and present educational systems? Have they given us a world free of ignorance, poverty, wars, crime and destruction?

The love or fear approach in teaching children determines their present and future. The way to acceptance and peace on earth begins as an inside job: inside each one of us, our social responsibility.

If you have major fear and stress surrounding the issues of education, health and your role in society, you may not see the options clearly. It is your responsibility to research and be informed of the best educational and health care you can find which fits within your belief systems. In this seminar, we will release fears concerning education as well as health issues such as: fear of illness, pain, fear of pain, doctors, operations, suffering, dying, and hospitals.

CAROL ANN HONTZ, B.S., M. ED., DD

Forty years in the field of education has taken Carol to many parts of the globe, first in public education, then Montessori Education and, since 1980, working in the field of spiritual, mental, physical and emotional health and wellness. She has been awarded The Most Outstanding Teacher Award from the University of New Jersey and The Distinguished Service to Humanity Award from Bloomsburg University of Pennsylvania, her Alma Maters. She is dedicated to the improvement of education for children and adults alike.

She is the President of Carol Kft., her Hungarian company; President of Carol Ann Hontz, International, Inc, owner of two Budapest Montessori Preschools; and founder of The Foundation for Integrated Education. She has taught Montessori teachers in Budapest and Prague, and was a sponsor of a number of Montessori Preschools and Elementary Schools in several Eastern European countries.

As a university student she traveled to France to study and later lived in Sicily, Venezuela, The Netherlands, The Czech Republic and Hungary, traveling extensively from these locations. While living in The Netherlands, Carol was introduced to specialized kinesiology (biofeedback/stress testing). The top American specialists in this field were teaching there. Among the many branches of specialized kinesiology she studied were Touch for Health, Educational Kinesiology, Behavioral Kinesiology, Applied Kinesiology, One Brain (where she is now Faculty Emeritus), Stress Release, and others. Teaching specialized kinesiology, she demonstrated her dedication to humanity, graduating 15,000 students in Russia, Poland, The Slovak and Czech Republics and Hungary since she began working there in 1991. Thousands of these students are now themselves working in this area, having their own centers and hundreds are teaching specialized kinesiology.

Carol developed and offers her series of courses for self-help and healing of the body, mind and spirit called "Metamorphosis". This system first identifies, and then corrects any specific negative emotion which can manifest itself in all forms of learning, relationship and health problems. The focus is that, as thinking is changed, energy changes. When that occurs, the body can heal itself very quickly, sometimes instantly, of dyslexia, allergies, phobias, addictions, obsessions, panic attacks, weight problems, eating disorders, and many other similar emotional and physical maladies.

A frequent guest on radio and television in Eastern Europe, Carol also gives many interviews to magazines and newspapers. She has authored two books: "Inner Treasures", "Infinite Potential". At a recent international conference for UNESCO, she lectured with top world scientists on Alternative Medicine. Earlier she lectured for an International UNESCO Peace Conference.

With thousands of students and clients changed in body, mind and spirit through her direct, personalized work and teaching, Carol has proven her techniques, best summarized in her "Metamorphosis" courses, to be an outstanding element in the area of Alternative Health Methods. With documented, impressive results, with her search for new and improved methodology, she continues to be a leader in this field.

Carol commutes between Europe and the USA where she is teaching, seeing clients and enjoying her family in the USA as well as her enormous international family.

For more information, refer to: www.carolannhontz.com